DIETARY RISK ASSESSMENT IN THE WIC PROGRAM

Committee on Dietary Risk Assessment
in the WIC Program

Food and Nutrition Board
INSTITUTE OF MEDICINE

NATIONAL ACADEMY PRESS
Washington, DC

NATIONAL ACADEMY PRESS • 2101 Constitution Avenue, N.W. • Washington, DC 20418

NOTICE: The project that is the subject of this report was approved by the Governing Board of the National Research Council, whose members are drawn from the councils of the National Academy of Sciences, the National Academy of Engineering, and the Institute of Medicine. The members of the committee responsible for the report were chosen for their special competences and with regard for appropriate balance.

Support for this project was provided by the Food and Nutrition Service, U.S. Department of Agriculture. The views presented in this report are those of the Institute of Medicine Committee on Dietary Risk Assessment in the WIC Program and are not necessarily those of the funding agency.

International Standard Book Number: 0-309-08284-6
Library of Congress Control Number: 2002100331

Additional copies of this report are available for sale from the National Academy Press, 2101 Constitution Avenue, N.W., Box 285, Washington, D.C. 20055. Call (800) 624-6242 or (202) 334-3313 (in the Washington metropolitan area), or visit the NAP's home page at **www.nap.edu**. The full text of this report is available at **www.nap.edu**.

For more information about the Institute of Medicine, visit the IOM home page at: **www.iom.edu**.

Copyright 2002 by the National Academy of Sciences. All rights reserved.

Printed in the United States of America.

The serpent has been a symbol of long life, healing, and knowledge among almost all cultures and religions since the beginning of recorded history. The serpent adopted as a logotype by the Institute of Medicine is a relief carving from ancient Greece, now held by the Staatliche Museen in Berlin.

Knowing is not enough; we must apply.
Willing is not enough; we must do.
—Goethe

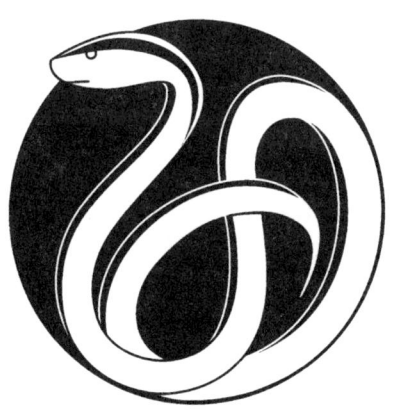

INSTITUTE OF MEDICINE

Shaping the Future for Health

THE NATIONAL ACADEMIES

National Academy of Sciences
National Academy of Engineering
Institute of Medicine
National Research Council

The **National Academy of Sciences** is a private, nonprofit, self-perpetuating society of distinguished scholars engaged in scientific and engineering research, dedicated to the furtherance of science and technology and to their use for the general welfare. Upon the authority of the charter granted to it by the Congress in 1863, the Academy has a mandate that requires it to advise the federal government on scientific and technical matters. Dr. Bruce M. Alberts is president of the National Academy of Sciences.

The **National Academy of Engineering** was established in 1964, under the charter of the National Academy of Sciences, as a parallel organization of outstanding engineers. It is autonomous in its administration and in the selection of its members, sharing with the National Academy of Sciences the responsibility for advising the federal government. The National Academy of Engineering also sponsors engineering programs aimed at meeting national needs, encourages education and research, and recognizes the superior achievements of engineers. Dr. Wm. A. Wulf is president of the National Academy of Engineering.

The **Institute of Medicine** was established in 1970 by the National Academy of Sciences to secure the services of eminent members of appropriate professions in the examination of policy matters pertaining to the health of the public. The Institute acts under the responsibility given to the National Academy of Sciences by its congressional charter to be an adviser to the federal government and, upon its own initiative, to identify issues of medical care, research, and education. Dr. Kenneth I. Shine is president of the Institute of Medicine.

The **National Research Council** was organized by the National Academy of Sciences in 1916 to associate the broad community of science and technology with the Academy's purposes of furthering knowledge and advising the federal government. Functioning in accordance with general policies determined by the Academy, the Council has become the principal operating agency of both the National Academy of Sciences and the National Academy of Engineering in providing services to the government, the public, and the scientific and engineering communities. The Council is administered jointly by both Academies and the Institute of Medicine. Dr. Bruce M. Alberts and Dr. Wm. A. Wulf are chairman and vice chairman, respectively, of the National Research Council.

COMMITTEE ON DIETARY RISK ASSESSMENT IN THE WIC PROGRAM

VIRGINIA A. STALLINGS (*chair*), Division of Gastroenterology and Nutrition, The Children's Hospital of Philadelphia, Pennsylvania

TOM BARANOWSKI, Department of Pediatrics, Baylor College of Medicine, Houston, Texas

RONETTE R. BRIEFEL, Mathematica Policy Research, Washington, D.C.

YVONNE BRONNER, Public Health Program, Morgan State University, Baltimore, Maryland

LAURA E. CAULFIELD, Department of International Health, Johns Hopkins University, Baltimore, Maryland

EZRA C. DAVIDSON, JR., Department of Obstetrics and Gynecology, Charles R. Drew University of Medicine and Science, Los Angeles, California

THERESA O. SCHOLL, Department of Obstetrics and Gynecology, University of Medicine and Dentistry of New Jersey, Stratford, New Jersey

CAROL W. SUITOR, Nutrition Consultant, Northfield, Vermont

ROBERT C. WHITAKER, Division of General and Community Pediatrics, Children's Hospital Medical Center, Cincinnati, Ohio

Staff

Romy Gunter-Nathan, Study Director
Kimberly Stitzel, Research Associate
Jaime Lanier, Project Assistant (until May 2001)
Peter Keo, Project Assistant (after May 2001)

FOOD AND NUTRITION BOARD

CUTBERTO GARZA (*chair*), Division of Nutritional Science, Cornell University, Ithaca, New York
ALFRED H. MERRILL, JR. (*vice chair*), School of Biology, Georgia Institute of Technology, Atlanta
ROBERT M. RUSSELL (*vice chair*), Jean Mayer U.S. Department of Agriculture Human Nutrition Research Center on Aging, Tufts University, Boston, Massachusetts
VIRGINIA A. STALLINGS (*vice chair*), Division of Gastroenterology and Nutrition, The Children's Hospital of Philadelphia, Pennsylvania
LARRY R. BEUCHAT, Center for Food Safety and Quality Enhancement, University of Georgia, Griffin
BENJAMIN CABALLERO, Center for Human Nutrition, Johns Hopkins Bloomberg School of Public Health, Baltimore, Maryland
ROBERT J. COUSINS, Center for Nutritional Sciences, University of Florida, Gainesville
SHIRIKI KUMANYIKA, Center for Clinical Epidemiology and Biostatistics, University of Pennsylvania School of Medicine, Philadelphia
LYNN PARKER, Child Nutrition Programs and Nutrition Policy, Food Research and Action Center, Washington, D.C.
ROSS L. PRENTICE, Division of Public Health Sciences, Fred Hutchinson Cancer Research Center, Seattle, Washington
A. CATHARINE ROSS, Department of Nutrition, The Pennsylvania State University, University Park
BARBARA O. SCHNEEMAN, Department of Nutrition, University of California, Davis
ROBERT E. SMITH, R.E. Smith Consulting, Inc., Newport, Vermont
STEVE L. TAYLOR, Food Processing Center, University of Nebraska, Lincoln
BARRY L. ZOUMAS, Department of Agricultural Economics and Rural Sociology, The Pennsylvania State University, University Park

Staff
ALLISON A. YATES, Director
LINDA D. MEYERS, Deputy Director
GAIL E. SPEARS, Administrative Assistant
GARY WALKER, Financial Associate

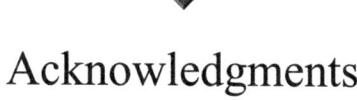

Acknowledgments

Sincere appreciation is extended to the many individuals and groups who were instrumental in the development of this report. First and foremost, many thanks are due to the committee members who volunteered countless hours to the research, deliberations, and preparation of the report. Their dedication to this project and to a stringent timeline was commendable, and the basis of our success.

Many individuals volunteered significant time and effort to address and educate our committee members during the workshop and public meeting. Workshop speakers included Jean Anliker, PhD, RD, University of Maryland; Ann Barone, LDN, Rhode Island Department of Health; Gladys Block, PhD, University of California at Berkeley; Graham Colditz, MD, DrPH, Harvard University; Cutberto Garza, MD, PhD, Cornell University; Bob Greenstein, Center on Budget and Policy Priorities, Washington, D.C.; Jill Leppert, LD, RD, North Dakota State Department of Health; Kristin Marcoe, MBA, RD, U.S. Department of Agriculture; Lynn Parker, MS, RD, Food Research and Action Center, Washington, D.C.; Carol Rankin, MS, RD, LD, Mississippi Department of Health; Anna Maria Siega-Riz, PhD, University of North Carolina; Amy Subar, PhD, MPH, RD, National Cancer Institute; Valerie Tarasuk, PhD, University of Toronto; and Amanda Watkins, MD, RD, Arizona Department of Health Services. In addition, two organizations provided oral testimony to the committee during its public meeting: the National Association of WIC Directors and the Food and Nutrition Service, U.S. Department of Agriculture. Sincere thanks and appreciation are also extended to Barbara Ainsworth, PhD, University of South

Carolina, for her valuable assistance as a consultant in the field of physical activity assessment.

This report has been reviewed in draft form by individuals chosen for their diverse perspectives and technical expertise, in accordance with procedures approved by the NRC's Report Review Committee. The purpose of this independent review is to provide candid and critical comments that will assist the institution in making its published report as sound as possible and to ensure that the report meets institutional standards for objectivity, evidence, and responsiveness to the study charge. The review comments and draft manuscript remain confidential to protect the integrity of the deliberative process. We wish to thank the following individuals for their review of this report:

Maxine Hayes, Washington State Department of Health
Jules Hirsch, Rockefeller University
Elvira Jarka, Health Resources and Services Administration
Louise C. Masse, National Cancer Institute
Esther Myers, American Dietetic Association
Valerie Tarasuk, University of Toronto

Although the reviewers listed above have provided many constructive comments and suggestions, they were not asked to endorse the conclusions or recommendations nor did they see the final draft of the report before its release. The review of this report was overseen by Gail Harrison, University of California, Los Angeles. Appointed by the National Research Council and Institute of Medicine, she was responsible for making certain that an independent examination of this report was carried out in accordance with institutional procedures and that all review comments were carefully considered. Responsibility for the final content of this report rests entirely with the authoring committee and the institution.

It is apparent that many organizations and individuals from a variety of clinical and scientific backgrounds provided timely and essential support for this project. Yet we would have never succeeded without the efforts, skills, and grace that was provided in large measure by Romy Gunter-Nathan, MPH, RD, our study director for this project; Kimberly Stitzel, MS, RD, research associate; Geraldine Kennedo, project assistant; Jaime Lanier, project assistant; Peter Keo, project assistant; and Allison A. Yates, PhD, RD, director, Food and Nutrition Board, Institute of Medicine.

Last, as chair, I express my sincere appreciation to each member of this committee for their extraordinary commitment to the project and the wonderful

ACKNOWLEDGMENTS

opportunity to work with them on this important task for the nutrition and policy community and for the women and children of the WIC population whose care we were asked to consider.

> Virginia A. Stallings, MD
> Chair, Committee on Dietary
> Risk Assessment in the WIC Program

Contents

EXECUTIVE SUMMARY 1

1 INTRODUCTION 13
    The WIC Program, 14
    Nutrition Risk Criteria, 15
    Dietary Risk, 19
    The Charge to the Committee and the Study Process, 22
    Organization of the Report, 24

2 DIETARY ASSESSMENT TOOLS IN WIC 27
    Purposes of Dietary Data Collection, 27
    Dietary Assessment Tools Currently Used by WIC Programs, 29
    Eligibility Criteria in Use, 32
    Summary, 33

3 USING THE *DIETARY GUIDELINES* AS THE BASIS OF
   DIETARY RISK CRITERIA 35
    The *Dietary Guidelines*, WIC, and National Goals, 35
    Which *Dietary Guidelines* Should be Targeted, 36

4 FRAMEWORK FOR EVALUATING TOOLS TO ASSESS
   DIETARY RISK 49
    Desirable Characteristics of an Assessment Tool, 49
    Summary, 55

5	FOOD-BASED ASSESSMENT OF DIETARY INTAKE 57
	A Focus on Usual Intake, 58
	Overview of Research-Quality Dietary Methods for Estimating Food or Nutrient Intake, 60
	Methods to Compare Food Intakes with the *Dietary Guidelines*, 79
	Conclusions Regarding Food-Based Dietary Assessment Methods for Eligibility Determination, 83
6	ASSESSMENT OF PHYSICAL ACTIVITY 85
	Challenges in Assessing Physical Activity, 85
	Methods to Assess Physical Activity, 88
	Conclusions Regarding the Role of Physical Activity Assessment for Eligibility Determination, 90
	Recommendations for Future Research, 92
7	BEHAVIORAL INDICATORS OF DIET AND PHYSICAL ACTIVITY 93
	The Concept of Behavioral Indicators, 94
	Behavioral Indicators of Diet, 96
	Behavioral Indicators of Physical Activity, 112
	Conclusions Regarding the Use of Behavioral Indicators for Eligibility Determination, 114
8	EVIDENCE OF DIETARY RISK AMONG LOW-INCOME WOMEN AND CHILDREN 115
	Nutritional Vulnerability of Groups Served by WIC, 115
	Results from Relevant Dietary Intake Studies, 120
	Associations of Food Intake with Income, 124
	Summary of Evidence Suggesting Dietary Risk, 126
9	FINDINGS AND RECOMMENDATIONS 129
	Findings, 129
	Recommendation, 133
	Concluding Remark, 135
10	REFERENCES 137

APPENDIXES
  A   Allowed Nutrition Risk Criteria, 159
  C   Workshop Agenda and Presentations, 163
  B   Biographical Sketches of Committee Members, 165

DIETARY RISK ASSESSMENT IN THE WIC PROGRAM

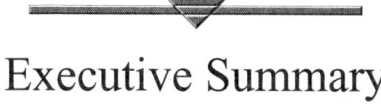

Executive Summary

Dietary intake patterns of individuals are complex in nature. However, assessing these complex patterns has been fundamental to the Special Supplemental Nutrition Program for Women, Infants, and Children (WIC) since its inception. The WIC program, which provides nutritious supplemental foods, nutrition education, and health referral services to low-income pregnant or postpartum women, infants, and children to age 5 years, requires applicants to meet one of several nutrition risk categories in order to be eligible for program services; dietary risk is one of these categories. Others include anthropometric risk (e.g., underweight, overweight), biochemical risk (e.g., low hematocrit), medical risk (e.g., diabetes mellitus), and other predisposing factors (e.g., homelessness). Since funds are not always available to meet the needs of the number of applicants determined to be eligible, a priority system is in place in which nutrition risk criteria are categorized based on severity of potential effect and outcome.

The role of dietary assessment in establishing eligibility for WIC is a crucial one, especially for postpartum women and children. As stated above, although eligibility may be based on many kinds of nutritional risks, substantial numbers of postpartum women and children currently are found to be eligible only on the basis of dietary risk. The practice of assessing dietary intake is widespread in part because, for those found to be at nutritional risk, the dietary data also influence the contents of the food package made available, nutrition education, and, sometimes, referrals. For this reason, even though many applicants are found to be at nutritional risk for a reason other than dietary risk, 86 percent of state agencies assess the dietary intake of all WIC participants. The practice consumes considerable time resources on the part of both WIC personnel and their clients.

In any venue, the assessment of dietary risk poses a challenge. Indeed, in an earlier report, the Institute of Medicine stated, "Research is urgently needed to develop practical and valid assessment tools for the identification of *inadequate diets*" (IOM, 1996). Moreover, a joint working group of the National Association of WIC Directors and of the Food and Nutrition Service of the U.S. Department of Agriculture did not find a sufficient scientific basis for developing standardized criteria for two major types of dietary risk: *failure to meet Dietary Guidelines* and *inadequate diet*. These are the two types of dietary risk that WIC personnel use extensively as the sole basis for determining that postpartum women and children are at nutritional risk.

Failure to meet Dietary Guidelines refers to the 10 guidelines in the *Dietary Guidelines for Americans* (USDA/HHS, 2000; see Box ES-1). These guidelines emphasize overall dietary and lifestyle patterns that can help to achieve favorable long-term health outcomes. Based on current knowledge about how dietary and physical activity patterns may reduce the risk of major chronic diseases and how a healthful diet may promote health, the 10 guidelines are designed to serve as the basis for federal policy and are used to guide nutrition information, education, and interventions for federal, state, and local agencies.

BOX ES-1 *Dietary Guidelines for Americans*

AIM FOR FITNESS...
- Aim for a healthy weight.
- Be physically active each day.

BUILD A HEALTHY BASE...
- Let the Pyramid guide your food choices.
- Choose a variety of grains daily, especially whole grains.
- Choose a variety of fruits and vegetables daily.
- Keep foods safe to eat.

CHOOSE SENSIBLY...
- Choose a diet that is low in saturated fat and cholesterol and moderate in total fat.
- Choose beverages and foods to moderate your intake of sugars.
- Choose and prepare foods with less salt.
- If you drink alcoholic beverages, do so in moderation.

SOURCE: USDA/HHS (2000).

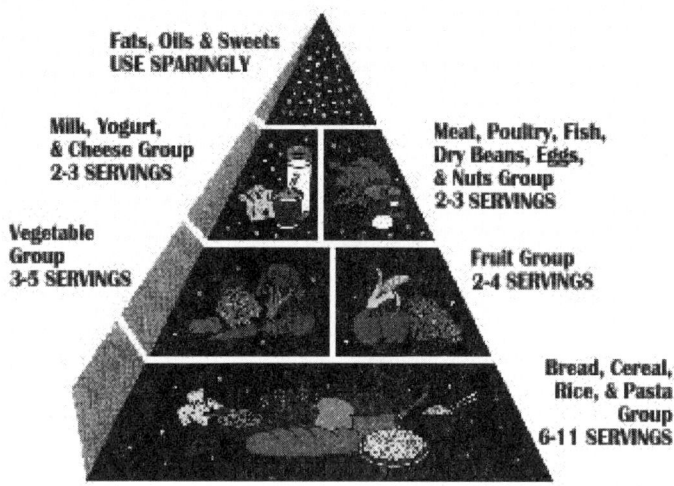

FIGURE ES-1 USDA Food Guide Pyramid.
SOURCE: USDA (1992).

Embedded in the guidelines is the Food Guide Pyramid—one of the major tools used for consumer nutrition education in the United States. The Pyramid (Figure ES-1) incorporates many of the *Dietary Guidelines* and gives concrete recommendations that promote moderation, balance, and variety in food intake.

THE TASK

Because of concern about the quality of dietary assessment methods and the resources in WIC required for using them to establish nutritional risk, the Food and Nutrition Service asked the Institute of Medicine (IOM) for assistance. In particular, it contracted with the IOM's Food and Nutrition Board to evaluate the use of various dietary assessment tools and to make recommendations for the assessment of inadequate or inappropriate dietary patterns, especially in the category *failure to meet Dietary Guidelines*. The Food and Nutrition Service asked that an expert committee propose a framework for assessing dietary risk among WIC applicants and identify and prioritize areas of greatest concern when the *Dietary Guidelines* are incorporated in WIC. In doing so, the committee was asked to focus on tools that could identify dietary risk of individuals accurately and thus be suitable for eligibility determination. The committee was also asked to recommend specific cut-off points for the criteria and to consider both food-based and behavior-based approaches. This report addresses those topics. However, since the *Dietary Guidelines* apply only to individuals ages 2 years and older, the focus is on pregnant and postpartum women and children.

CURRENT PRACTICES

Since standardized criteria have not yet been established for *failure to meet Dietary Guidelines* or *inadequate diets*, state WIC agencies currently select the method and cut-off points to be used by their agencies. The most commonly used methods are 24-hour diet recalls and food frequency questionnaires. WIC personnel generally compare dietary intake data obtained using one or both of these methods with specified numbers of servings from each of the five basic food groups of the Food Guide Pyramid. In most cases, the methods used appear not to have undergone studies of accuracy or reliability. Many state WIC agencies use the Food Guide Pyramid servings as a standard for children ages 12 to 24 months even though the Pyramid was designed for persons ages 2 years and older.

A FRAMEWORK FOR ASSESSING DIETARY RISK

In an interim report (IOM, 2000c), the Committee on Dietary Risk Assessment in the WIC Program proposed a framework that consists of eight characteristics essential to a food-based and/or behavior-based tool designed for eligibility determination. That framework has been modified slightly in this report. An optimal tool should:

- use specific criteria that are related to health or disease;
- be appropriate for age and physiological condition (e.g., pregnancy or lactation);
- serve three purposes: screening for eligibility, tailoring of food packages,[1] and nutrition education;
- have acceptable performance characteristics (validity and reliability);
- be suitable for the culture and language of the population served;
- be responsive to operational constraints in the WIC setting;
- be standardized across states/agencies; and
- allow prioritization within the category of dietary risk.

The committee considered these characteristics as it examined possible methods for determining dietary risk.

---

[1] The types and amounts of foods in WIC food packages may be adjusted somewhat to accommodate a participant's particular nutritional needs or food preferences.

TABLE ES-1 Recommended Number of Pyramid Servings by Physiologic Status/Energy Intake and Food Group

Food Group	Children Ages 2–3 yr ($\approx$ 1,300 kcal)	Children Ages 4–6 yr, Women ($\approx$1,600 kcal)	Moderately Active Women, Some Pregnant Women ($\approx$1,800 kcal)	Teen Girls; Active, Pregnant, or Lactating Women ($\approx$ 2,200 kcal)
Grains group, especially whole grain	6	6	7	9
Vegetable group	3	3	3.3	4
Fruit group	2	2	2.3	3
Milk group, preferably fat free or low fat	2[a]	2 or 3[b]	2 or 3[b]	2 or 3[b]
Meat and beans group, preferably lean or low fat	2	2, for a total of 5 oz	2, for a total of 6 oz	2, for a total of 6 oz

[a]Portion sizes are reduced for children ages 2–3 years, except for milk.
[b]The number of servings from the milk group depends on age. Older children and teenagers (ages 9 to 18 years) need three servings daily. Women 19 years and older need two servings daily. During pregnancy and lactation, the recommended number of milk group servings is the same as for nonpregnant females of the same age.

SOURCE: Adapted from USDA/HHS (2000).

FINDINGS AND RECOMMENDATION

Findings

Basing Risk Criteria on the Dietary Guidelines

Focusing on the single guideline *Let the Pyramid Guide Your Food Choices* was determined to be the most feasible, comprehensive, and objective approach to using the *Dietary Guidelines* for establishing dietary risk for those individuals 2 years of age and older. Based on review of the *Dietary Guidelines* and the scientific underpinnings of the Food Guide Pyramid, the committee determined that this approach should use the recommended number of servings based on energy needs as the cut-off point for each of the five basic food groups (see Table ES-1). For example, the criterion for active, pregnant, adult women would be at least nine servings from the grains group. A majority of state WIC agencies already use some version of this approach as the basis for setting a criterion that addresses the dietary risk *failure to meet Dietary Guidelines*.

Finding 1. A dietary risk criterion that uses the WIC applicant's usual intake of the five basic Pyramid food groups as the indicator and the recommended numbers of servings based on energy needs as the cut-off points is consistent with *failure to meet Dietary Guidelines.*

Prevalence of Dietary Risk Based on the Food Guide Pyramid Recommendations

More than 96 percent of individuals in the United States, and an even higher percentage of low-income individuals (such as those served by WIC), do not usually consume the recommended number of servings specified by the Food Guide Pyramid (Krebs-Smith et al., 1997; Munoz et al., 1997). Thus, the identification of individuals who are *not* at dietary risk becomes highly problematic.

Finding 2. Nearly all U.S. women and children usually consume fewer than the recommended number of servings specified by the Food Guide Pyramid and, therefore, would be at dietary risk based on the criterion *failure to meet Dietary Guidelines* that is described in Finding 1.

Food-Based Assessment of Dietary Intake

Nutritional status and health are influenced by usual or long-term dietary intake. For this reason, dietary assessment for establishing WIC eligibility should be based on usual intake. Day-to-day variation in food and nutrient intake by individuals is so large in the United States that one or two 24-hour diet recalls or food records cannot provide accurate information about an individual's usual intake. In the WIC setting, it is impractical to obtain more than one or two recalls or records under standardized conditions that would promote accurate reporting. Moreover, most people make many errors when reporting their food intake because of the complex nature of the task. These errors increase the likelihood that eligibility status for WIC will be misclassified in the category of dietary risk.

Food frequency questionnaires (FFQs) are designed to assess usual intake and may be practical to administer to many WIC clients. However, they are subject to many types of errors, and their performance characteristics are unsatisfactory for determining individual eligibility. For example, when reported food or nutrient intakes from an FFQ are compared with the values obtained using a large number of research-quality diet recalls or food records, correlations generally range between 0.3 and 0.7. Although correlations in that range may be considered satisfactory for making inferences about intakes by groups of individuals in epidemiologic research, such data cannot accurately classify individuals as above or below set cut-off points—a serious problem when the goal is determining the eligibility of an individual. Shortening FFQs generally makes them more responsive to operational constraints, but further reduces their accuracy and utility.

Few practical methods have been developed or tested that compare food intakes with the *Dietary Guidelines* or Food Guide Pyramid recommendations. Such methods would require converting amounts of each type of food consumed to Pyramid portions to determine whether the Food Guide Pyramid recommendations had been met. This is a complex process, especially for mixed dishes, and does not lend itself to operational constraints in the WIC setting.

> **Finding 3.** Even research-quality dietary assessment methods are not sufficiently accurate or precise to distinguish an individual's eligibility status using criteria based on the Food Guide Pyramid or on nutrient intake.

Physical Activity Assessment

Because the committee was asked to identify areas of concern when the *Dietary Guidelines* were incorporated into WIC and because the *Guidelines* include a quantitative recommendation for physical activity levels for adults and for children 2 years of age and older, the committee considered physical activity assessment as a part of dietary risk assessment. Although a physical activity recommendation appears in the *Dietary Guidelines*, physical activity itself is not currently part of dietary risk assessment in WIC, nor is there a separate nutritional risk criterion in the WIC program related to physical activity. However, given that (1) WIC's mandate is to focus on primary prevention, including the primary prevention of overweight and obesity, (2) the increasing degree to which overweight and obesity are now major health concerns among those served by WIC, and (3) proper risk assessment for prevention or treatment must consider both diet and physical activity, it is likely that WIC may soon consider assessing physical activity, even if not for the purposes of eligibility determination.

Physical activity assessment relates to two of the *Dietary Guidelines* (*Aim For A Healthy Weight* and *Be Physically Active Each Day*) and thus could potentially be used as another way to define *failure to meet Dietary Guidelines*. The physical activity guideline specifies "Aim to accumulate at least 30 minutes (adults) or 60 minutes (children) of moderate physical activity most days of the week, preferably daily." These specifications could be used as WIC eligibility criteria under the dietary risk subgroup *failure to meet Dietary Guidelines*.

A review of the literature found no physical activity assessment instruments that meet the operational constraints of WIC and that also can accurately and reliably assess whether a woman or child is obtaining at least the specified amount of physical activity. Because of the inherent cognitive challenge of accurately recalling and characterizing the varied activity behaviors that together constitute an individual's physical activity level, it is unlikely that there could ever be a practical instrument to establish WIC eligibility accurately based on the physical activity recommendation in the *Dietary Guidelines*.

> **Finding 4.** Physical activity assessment methods are not sufficiently accurate or reliable to distinguish individuals who are ineligible from those who are eligible for WIC services based on the physical activity component of the *Dietary Guidelines*.

Behavioral Indicators of Diet and Physical Activity

Because certain behaviors are correlated with dietary intake and physical activity, interest has arisen in the use of behavior-based assessment as a method of identifying those who usually fail to meet the *Dietary Guidelines*. Such assessment would require the identification of behavioral indicators that could distinguish individuals who meet the *Dietary Guidelines* from those who do not. The committee considered two types of behavioral indicators: surrogate and target. Surrogate behaviors are behaviors that are correlated with one or more aspects of diet or physical activity and could be used to make inferences about what children eat or how much activity they engage in. For example, the frequency of eating meals together as a family could indicate the adequacy of vegetable consumption. Target behaviors are behaviors that make good targets for change. Making changes in a target behavior would be expected to result in changes in dietary intake. Target behavioral indicators are not suitable for eligibility determination unless they also are surrogate indicators. Building on the example above, if families could be encouraged to eat meals together more frequently, and if family meals resulted in improved dietary intake, then frequency of eating meals as a family would be both a surrogate indicator and a potential target indicator for change. By analogy, if families could spend more time outdoors and if this change resulted in increased levels of physical activity, then time spent outdoors could be both a surrogate and target indicator for physical activity.

A review of the literature found few studies of behavioral correlates of diet or physical activity conducted among the groups served by WIC. No strong evidence was found that any examined behaviors would be both adequately reliable and accurate as surrogate or target behavioral indicators.

Finding 5. Behavioral indicators have weak relationships with dietary or physical activity outcomes of interest. As a result, they hold no promise of distinguishing individuals who are ineligible for WIC from those who are eligible in the category of dietary risk.

Recommendation

Based on the above findings, the following recommendation is made:

> **Presume that all women and children (ages 2 to 5 years) who meet the eligibility requirements of income, categorical, and residency status also meet the requirement of nutrition risk through the category of dietary risk based on *failure to meet Dietary Guidelines*, where *failure to meet Dietary Guidelines* is defined as consuming fewer than the recommended number of servings from one or more of the five basic food groups (grains, fruits, vegetables, milk products, and meat or beans) based on an individual's estimated energy needs.**

Studies suggest that nearly all women in the childbearing years and children ages 2 years and older are at dietary risk because they fail to meet the *Dietary Guidelines* as translated by recommendations of the Food Guide Pyramid (Krebs-Smith et al., 1997; Munoz et al., 1997) (See Table ES-1 for the recommended number of servings based on an individual's energy needs.) Tools currently used for dietary risk assessment appear to have very high sensitivity in that they identify nearly everyone as failing to meet the *Dietary Guidelines*, but low specificity—poor ability to identify persons who are not at dietary risk. No known dietary or physical activity assessment methods or behavioral indicators of diet or physical activity hold promise of accurately identifying the small percentage of women and children who do meet the proposed criterion based on the Food Guide Pyramid or the physical activity recommendation. Even if the percentage of individuals who meet the criterion were to increase substantially, it remains unlikely that methods can be found or developed to differentiate risk among individuals.

When WIC was originally established in 1972, the categorical groups that WIC serves were selected because of their vulnerability to nutritional insults and WIC's potential for preventing nutrition-related problems. Nutritional status and dietary intake have both short- and long-term effects on the health of the woman and on the growth, development, and health of the fetus, infant, or child. The groups served by WIC also are at increased risk of morbidity and mortality from virtually every disorder listed among the leading causes of death in the United

States (cardiovascular disease, cancer, diabetes, and digestive diseases). The high prevalence of overweight and obesity and of diets that are inconsistent with the *Dietary Guidelines* (e.g., low intakes of fruits and vegetables, high intakes of saturated fats) may contribute to these increased risks.

This recommendation is not intended to affect the current use of other nutritional risk criteria for eligibility determination. That is, information should continue to be collected for the identification of other nutrition risks (e.g., hemoglobin or hematocrit to identify risk of anemia, height and weight to identify anthropometric risk, and the presence of diabetes mellitus to identify medical risk). Such information is useful for nutrition education, and it is essential to implement the priority system. When funds are insufficient to enroll all those eligible for WIC, the priority system is used to determine those at greatest need. If dietary information is collected in the WIC setting for food package tailoring, nutrition education, and/or health referrals, the methods used should be approached with caution given the likelihood of error and misclassification.

Optimal Collection and Use of Dietary and Physical Activity Data

Although individual-level reporting errors greatly reduce the validity of data for assessing diet or physical activity levels in individuals, the errors are less serious in group assessments. Moreover, a variety of statistical procedures can adjust for known sources of error (IOM, 2000a; Traub, 1994) and thereby provide reasonable tests of relationships. Thus, while identified relationships may not be true for any specific individual, they would be true for the group. For example, FFQs and diet recalls can be used to identify dietary patterns in a WIC population and patterns needing improvement. Repeated collection of dietary recalls or FFQs also may be used to monitor change over time at the group level or to assess effects of nutrition education interventions.

Findings from such analyses could be used to design nutrition education programs and monitor their effectiveness. For example, diet recalls can provide valid information on the average intakes of groups, assuming that a standardized data collection approach is used and an adequate sample size (50 or larger) is available. If more than one recall is collected on at least a subsample of the group and appropriate adjustments are made, one could determine the proportion of the group with usual nutrient intakes that are less than the Estimated Average Requirement (IOM, 2000a). Group dietary intake information for a WIC population (e.g., data from a recent national dietary survey such as the National Health and Nutrition Examination Survey or the Continuing Survey of Food Intakes by Individuals or data collected in a special WIC study) could be used to identify areas for targeted nutrition education services.

Likewise, physical activity assessment tools may be sufficiently valid to assess physical activity levels within groups. These data would be valuable for monitoring groups of individuals or "target populations" within WIC that may be at higher risk for low physical activity levels and/or that may benefit most from interventions within WIC to increase physical activity levels.

Group assessment data would best be collected by trained individuals on randomly selected subsamples of the WIC population. However, any tool used for this purpose must still be evaluated in terms of desired criteria (e.g., a tool would still need to be easy to administer, appropriate for the group, and reasonably accurate).

CONCLUDING REMARK

In summary, evidence exists to conclude that nearly all low-income women in the childbearing years and children ages 2 to 5 years are at dietary risk, are vulnerable to nutrition insults, and may benefit from WIC's services. Further, due to the complex nature of dietary patterns, it is unlikely that a tool will be developed to fulfill its intended purpose within WIC: to classify individuals accurately with respect to their true dietary risk. Thus, any tools adopted would result in misclassification of the eligibility status of some, potentially many, individuals. By presuming that all who meet the categorical and income eligibility requirements are at dietary risk, WIC retains its potential for preventing and correcting nutrition-related problems while avoiding serious misclassification errors that could lead to denial of services to eligible individuals.

1

Introduction

The Special Supplemental Nutrition Program for Women, Infants, and Children (WIC) provides supplemental foods, nutrition education, and health referral services to low-income pregnant or postpartum women, infants, and young children. As specified in the Child Nutrition Act of 1966, the program is intended to "serve as an adjunct to good health care, during critical times of growth and development; to prevent the occurrence of health problems, including drug abuse; and improve the health status of these persons" (Child Nutrition Act of 1966 [As Amended Through Public Law 106-224, June 20, 2000]). The program is based on the premise that low income predisposes women, infants, and children to poor nutritional status and adverse health outcomes. Part of establishing program eligibility (see later section, "Nutrition Risk Criteria") requires the determination of nutritional risk. By identifying individuals with specific nutrition-related risks and providing food and services targeted at reducing these risks, the program seeks to improve overall health and birth outcomes.

Dietary risk is only one of five categories of nutrition risk, but it is the basis for WIC eligibility for a large percentage of applicants. However, methods for identifying individuals who are at dietary risk have posed a long-standing problem for this program. This report seeks to evaluate the use of various dietary assessment tools and to make recommendations for their use in identifying individuals who are at dietary risk. It focuses on two types of dietary risk: *failure to meet Dietary Guidelines* and *inadequate diet*.

THE WIC PROGRAM

Established in 1972 through an amendment to the Child Nutrition Act of 1966, the WIC program has grown substantially and in 2001 served about 7.3 million participants each month (USDA, 2001d). The program is administered by the Food and Nutrition Service (FNS) of the U.S. Department of Agriculture (USDA). In fiscal year 2000, FNS provided cash grants totaling $4.1 billion to 88 state agencies (USDA, 2000a). State agencies include all 50 states, the 5 U.S. Territories (American Samoa, the District of Columbia, Guam, Puerto Rico, and the American Virgin Islands), and 33 Indian Tribal Organizations. Together, state agencies administer the WIC program through approximately 2,000 local WIC agencies and 10,000 service sites (USDA, 2001b).

Unlike the Food Stamp or Medicaid Programs, WIC is not an entitlement program. Rather, it is a grant program for which funding limits are set annually by Congress. Like some other federal programs, WIC requires applicants to meet income and categorical criteria (in this case, pregnant, postpartum, or lactating women and children under the age of 5 years). WIC is unique, however, in that applicants also must be found to have a nutrition risk to be eligible for participation. Nutrition risk categories include anthropometric, biochemical, medical, and dietary risks, as well as some predisposing conditions (see Box 1-1

BOX 1-1 WIC Eligibility Requirements

Categorical Status	Applicants must fall into one of the following categories:
	Women:
	    Pregnant or up to 6 weeks following the birth of an infant or at the end of the pregnancy
	    Postpartum (up to 6 months after the birth of the infant or the end of the pregnancy)
	    Breastfeeding (up to the infant's first birthday)
	Infants:
	    Up to the infant's first birthday
	Children:
	    From first birthday up to the child's fifth birthday

Income Level	Applicants must have an income level at or below 185 percent of the federal poverty level or be adjunctively eligible through enrollment in Medicaid, temporary assistance to needy families, or the Food Stamp program
Residency	Applicants must live in the state in which they apply
Nutrition Risk	Applicants must be determined to be at nutrition risk (e.g., Anthropometric, Medical, Dietary, or Predisposing Conditions [see Box 1-3])

SOURCE: USDA (2001c).

for a summary of WIC eligibility requirements). The categorical and nutrition risk categories provide a means to prioritize individuals based on health risk and the potential to benefit from the program. Such prioritization is necessary when funding is not sufficient to provide benefits to all who meet the categorical and income eligibility requirements. In recent years, funding has been sufficient to eliminate essentially all waiting lists. However, if prioritization were necessary because of limited funding, services would be offered according to a seven-level priority system (Box 1-2).

NUTRITION RISK CRITERIA

Nutritional risk is composed of five broad categories: anthropometric, biochemical, clinical/health/medical, dietary, or other. Each of these categories contains

---

BOX 1-2 WIC Priority System

Priority	
I	Pregnant women, breastfeeding women, and infants at nutritional risk as demonstrated by hematological or anthropometric measurements, or other documented nutritionally related medical conditions which demonstrate the need for supplemental foods.
II	Except those infants who qualify for Priority I, infants up to 6 months of age born of program participants who participated during pregnancy, and infants up to 6 months of age born of women who were not Program participants during pregnancy but whose medical records document that they were at nutritional risk during pregnancy due to nutritional conditions detectable by biochemical or anthropometric measurements or other documented nutritionally related medical conditions which demonstrated the person's need for supplemental foods.
III	Children at nutritional risk as demonstrated by hematological or anthropometric measurements or other documented medical conditions that demonstrate the child's need for supplemental foods.
IV	Pregnant women, breastfeeding women, and infants at nutritional risk because of an inadequate dietary pattern.
V	Children at nutritional risk because of inadequate dietary pattern.
VI	Postpartum women at nutritional risk.
VII	Individuals certified for WIC solely due to homelessness or migrancy and, at State agency option, and in accordance with the provisions of paragraph (e)(1)(iii) of this section, previously certified participants who might regress in nutritional status without continued provision of supplemental foods.

SOURCE: 7 C.F.R. Subpart C, Section 246.7(e)(4).

subgroups of indicators and specific criteria. A criterion is defined as a nutrition risk indicator and its cut-off point. For example, *elevated blood lead level* is a biochemical indicator. The approved criterion is a blood lead value greater than or equal to 10 µg/dL. Box 1-3 lists the five broad categories of nutrition risk criteria and their most common subgroups. A complete list of currently approved nutrition risk criteria can be found in Appendix A.

A history of dietary risk assessment in the WIC program provides a useful background for the current study (see Box 1-4). Until recently, state agencies had been permitted to develop their own nutrition risk criteria using broad federal guidelines. As expected, this flexibility resulted in wide variation for indicators and cut-offs. In 1989, prompted by concern over the variation in eligibility determination, Congress mandated a review of the nutrition risk criteria and priority system. In 1993, FNS contracted with the Food and Nutrition Board (FNB) of the Institute of Medicine (IOM), National Academies, to conduct a comprehensive scientific assessment of the nutrition risk criteria for use as eligibility criteria in the WIC program.

In 1996, IOM released its recommendations through the report *WIC Nutrition Risk Criteria: A Scientific Assessment* (IOM, 1996). With regard to dietary risk, the report reviewed three major categories: inappropriate dietary patterns, inadequate diet, and food insecurity. Documenting clear health and nutrition risks associated with selected inappropriate dietary patterns, the report concluded that individuals at risk for these patterns have a high potential to benefit from participation in the WIC program. It recommended the development of valid assessment tools for the purpose of identifying commonly consumed foods, thereby providing a starting point for nutrition education. With regard to *inadequate diet* as an eligibility criterion, the committee recommended discontinuing its use as a criterion for eligibility. With regard to food insecurity, the committee concluded that those at risk would likely benefit from participation in the WIC program. However, while the committee recommended that food insecurity be included as a risk criterion, they found insufficient scientific evidence on which to select a cut-off point to identify those most likely to benefit.

USDA has made progress in the development of tools to assess food security since the 1996 IOM report's recommendation to include food insecurity as a criterion. In particular, USDA has developed an 18-item assessment form and supported the development of a 6-item short form by Blumberg and colleagues for use in measuring household food security (Blumberg et al., 1999). Some WIC clinics use similar instruments or include food security questions in their client interviews. However, there currently are no available tools that accurately assess food insecurity at the individual level.

Food insecurity is associated with a higher risk of an inadequate diet and is strongly related to household income, but individuals living in food secure households can still have inadequate diets. The committee recognizes the

> **BOX 1-3** Categories and Subgroups of Nutritional Risk Criteria Developed by the National Association of WIC Directors
>
> **Anthropometric**
> - Low weight for height
> - High weight for height
> - Short stature
> - Inappropriate growth/weight gain pattern
> - Low birth weight/premature birth
> - Other anthropometric risk
>
> **Biochemical**
> - Hematocrit or hemoglobin below state criteria
> - Other biochemical test results which indicate nutritional abnormality (such as cholesterol, folic acid, vitamin B_6, vitamin B_{12}, other nutritional anemias)
>
> **Clinical/Health/Medical**
> - Pregnancy-induced conditions (such as toxemia, preeclampsia, eclampsia, pregnancy-induced hypertension, gestational diabetes, excessive vomiting, and nausea)
> - Delivery of low-birth weight/premature infant
> - Prior stillbirth, miscarriage, spontaneous abortion, or neonatal death
> - General obstetrical risks (such as multiple fetus births, high parity, closely spaced pregnancies, age)
> - Nutrition-related risk conditions (such as any nutrition-related chronic disease, genetic disorder, infectious disease, clinical malnutrition, failure to thrive, drug–nutrient interactions)
> - Substance abuse (drugs, alcohol, tobacco)
> - Other health risk (mental retardation, for example)
>
> **Dietary**
> - Inadequate/inappropriate nutrient intake
> - Other dietary risk
>
> **Other Risk**
> - Regression
> - Transfer (nutrition risk unknown)
> - Breastfeeding mother/infant dyad
> - Infant of a WIC-eligible mother or mother at risk during pregnancy
> - Homelessness/migrancy
> - Other nutritional risks
>
> SOURCE: USDA (2001c).

significance of food insecurity as a potential contributing factor to dietary risk and nutritional risk, but it did not specifically address the question of assessing food insecurity within the WIC population for several reasons: (1) the available

BOX 1-4 History of Dietary Risk Assessment in the WIC Program

1974	The Special Supplemental Nutrition Program for Women, Infants, and Children (WIC) was established through an amendment to the Child Nutrition Act of 1966.
1975	Regulatory requirements defined Dietary Risk as "known inadequate nutritional patterns."
1976	Regulatory requirements established minimum data collection to establish nutrition risk. The requirements included the collection of anthropometric, biochemical, diet history, and 24-hour recall data.
1978	Nutrition risk was defined by legislative authority as "Dietary deficiencies that impair or endanger health, such as inadequate dietary patterns assessed by a 24-hour recall, dietary history, or food frequency checklist."
1985	A General Accounting Office report suggested the need to refine dietary assessment methodology to make more reliable measures of nutritional risk and to increase uniformity in assessment across states.
1990	Congress mandated a review of nutrition risk criteria and the priority system through Public Law 101-147. The Task Force on Dietary Assessment was established to identify dietary assessment methodologies applicable to the WIC program. It recommended the use of a food frequency instrument.
1991	The Harvard Cooperative Agreement developed a Food Frequency Questionnaire (FFQ), but it was not validated in the WIC population.
1993	FNS contracted with IOM to conduct a comprehensive scientific assessment of the nutrition risk criteria for use as eligibility criteria.
1994	The WIC Dietary Assessment Validation Study evaluated two sets of FFQs (Harvard and Block) for potential use in screening African-American, Hispanic, or white women and children for eligibility in the WIC program. Using a cut-off of less than 100 percent of the RDA was found to qualify virtually all income-eligible women and children.
1996	IOM released recommendations through the report, *WIC Nutrition Risk Criteria: A Scientific Assessment*.
1998	The Risk Identification and Selection Collaborative (RISC) was established to conduct an ongoing review of nutrition risk criteria (January 21, 1998). Policy Memorandum 98-9 was released by FNS for review by state agencies. The memorandum contained lists of nutrition risk criteria that were either (a) approved for certification; (b) not approved for certification; or (c) referred to RISC for further deliberations.
1999	WIC agencies began using only approved nutrition risk criteria for WIC certification (April 1, 1999). USDA contracted with IOM to review the scientific basis for methods currently employed in the assessment of individuals for eligibility to the WIC program based on dietary risk.

measurement tool is an income-driven assessment at the household level rather than a dietary risk assessment at the individual level; (2) while food insecurity is considered to be one of several factors that could potentially put an individual at dietary risk, it is not an accurate indicator of all those at dietary risk; and (3) it falls outside the specific definitions of *failure to meet Dietary Guidelines* and *inadequate diet.*

Following the release of the 1996 IOM report, FNS and the National Association of WIC Directors (NAWD) formed a joint working group, the Risk Identification and Selection Collaborative (RISC), to address recommendations of the IOM report and to develop standardized and scientifically sound nutrition risk criteria. The intent was to achieve greater consistency among state and local WIC agencies. Through multiple subcommittees, the RISC working group developed three lists of nutrition risk criteria: criteria that are allowed, criteria that are not allowed, and criteria that are in need of future review. FNS released a final policy memorandum in June 1998 that described over 100 allowable nutrition risk criteria. These criteria were implemented as of April 1, 1999 (FNS, 1998), and continue to be updated regularly. The current list of allowable criteria can be found in Appendix A. In order to allow states some flexibility to meet local priorities and needs, state agencies may establish more restrictive cut-off points as long as definitions of the indicators are not changed. For example, a state may choose to use "greater than the ninety-fifth percentile of weight for height" rather than the cut off of the nineteth percentile cited in the allowable risk criterion (FNS, 1998).

DIETARY RISK

The focus of this report falls within one category of nutrition risk: dietary risk. More specifically, it focuses on methods or tools used to assess risk of an individual according to two specific dietary risk criteria: *failure to meet Dietary Guidelines* and *inadequate diet.*

Data from state agencies make it clear that dietary risk is the most commonly reported nutrition risk in WIC applicants—no other single category comes close. In 1998, 49 percent of WIC applicants (47 percent of women, 13 percent of infants, and 68 percent of children ages 1 to 5 years) were reported to have met dietary risk criteria (Bartlett et al., 2000). Because of differences in reporting practices, these percentages are likely to be underestimated. The second most commonly reported subcategory of nutrition risk was "high weight for height," at 17 percent of participants. Again, because of differences in reporting practices, this percentage is likely to be underestimated. Only two-thirds of state agencies report all documented risk criteria for participants; the remaining third follow some other type of reporting procedure (e.g., they report only the three or four most serious nutrition risks).

The percentage of children served by WIC found to be at dietary risk has increased steadily over the years. In 1992, 52 percent of WIC-served children were reported to be at dietary risk compared to 68 percent in 1998 (Bartlett et al., 2000). A portion of this increase reflects the growth of WIC—increased funding allowed WIC to serve more children in priority level 5 (Box 1-2).

Defining Dietary Risk

As defined by the Code of Federal Regulations, dietary risk refers to dietary deficiencies that impair or endanger health, such as inadequate dietary patterns assessed by a 24-hour dietary recall, dietary history, or food frequency checklist (7CFR Subpart C, Section 246.7(e)(2)(iii)). WIC eligibility based on this category is intended to prevent the occurrence of malnutrition or other overt problems of dietary origin due to suboptimal dietary patterns, and result in improved health outcomes for the pregnant woman, mother, fetus, infant, and young child.

Most states generally define dietary risk as failure to consume a minimum number of servings from one or more food groups represented in the Food Guide Pyramid (see Chapter 2). The 1996 IOM report defined dietary inadequacy as food or nutrient intake insufficient to meet a specified percentage of the Recommended Dietary Allowances (RDAs) (NRC, 1989) for one or more nutrients (IOM, 1996). Determination of *inadequate diet* has historically involved estimating nutrient intakes using some method of dietary recall or food frequency questionnaire and then comparing the reported intake with a specified percentage of the RDAs for the individual (often between 70 and 100 percent of the RDA) (IOM, 1996).

WIC Policy Memorandum 98-9 contains 18 specific dietary risk criteria (Box 1-5). Although state agencies may only use criteria on the allowable list, the agencies are given the prerogative to exclude an allowable criteria if so desired. Although *failure to meet Dietary Guidelines* (401) and *inadequate diet* (422) are included among the 18 allowable dietary risk criteria, they are the only two for which definitions and cut-off points have not been set officially. State agencies continue to be accorded discretion within broad federal guidelines to define these two criteria (the indicators and cut-off points to be used) and choose tools to assess them.

Early in the study, the committee recognized confusion with the terms used to describe dietary risk—specifically inadequate and inappropriate diets or patterns. For this reason, the committee adopted working definitions for use in this report. *Dietary risk* is a broad term and refers to any inappropriate dietary pattern. *Inappropriate dietary pattern* includes both *inadequate* and *excessive* intakes of food, nutrients, or other dietary substances over time that are unsuit- able for optimal health, growth, or development according to the *Dietary Guidelines for Americans* (*Dietary Guidelines*) (USDA/HHS, 2000). It also includes other

> **BOX 1-5** Dietary Risk Assessment Indicators Allowed for WIC Program Certification
>
> 400 Inadequate/Inappropriate Nutrient Intake
>   401 Failure to meet Dietary Guidelines
>   402 Vegan Diets
>   403 Highly Restrictive Diets
> 410 Other Dietary Risk
>   411 Inappropriate Infant Feeding
>   412 Early Introduction of Solid Foods
>   413 Feeding Cow's Milk During First 12 Months
>   414 No Dependable Source of Iron for Full-Term Infants at 6 Months of Age or Later
>   415 Improper Dilution of Formula
>   416 Feeding Other Foods Low in Essential Nutrients
>   417 Lack of Sanitation in Preparation/Handling of Nursing Bottles
>   418 Infrequent Breastfeeding as Sole Source of Nutrients
>   419 Inappropriate Use of Nursing Bottles
>   420 Excessive Caffeine Intake (Breastfeeding Woman)
>   421 Pica
>   422 Inadequate Diet
>   423 Inappropriate or Excessive Intake of Dietary Supplements Including Vitamins, Minerals, and Herbal Remedies
>   424 Inadequate Vitamin/Mineral Supplementation
>   425 Inappropriate Feeding Practices for Children
>
> SOURCE: Food and Nutrition Service (FNS, 1998).

undesirable patterns or practices (e.g., early introduction of solid foods to infants, feeding cow's milk before age 1 year).

- *Inadequate dietary intake* is a subgroup of inappropriate dietary patterns and refers to dietary intake that is either low in nutrients (inadequate nutrient intake) or low in food group servings as specified in the *Dietary Guidelines* (see Chapter 4).
- *Excessive dietary intake* is a subgroup of inappropriate dietary patterns and refers to overconsumption of energy, nutrients, or food group servings as specified in the *Dietary Guidelines*).

The committee viewed these descriptors as overlapping rather than as discreet entities. For example, dietary intake that meets the definition of *inadequate diet* would also meet the definition of inappropriate diet or *failure to meet*

Dietary Guidelines. However, a diet that meets the definition for *failure to meet Dietary Guidelines* would not necessarily meet the definition for *inadequate diet*.

History of the Indicator *Failure to Meet Dietary Guidelines*

The 1996 IOM report documented evidence to support the use of *Dietary patterns that fail to meet the Dietary Guidelines* as an indicator of both health risk and benefit in the WIC program. Consequently, it recommended the use of the 1995 *Dietary Guidelines* (USDA/HHS, 1995) in setting dietary risk criteria for women and for children over 2 years of age. However, the report did not provide guidance about how to do so. Instead, it noted that "any cut-off points would be arbitrary," and recommended "research to develop and test practical dietary assessment instruments that would identify those who fail to meet Dietary Guidelines" (IOM, 1996).

Since the release of the IOM report's recommendation in 1996, the *Dietary Guidelines* have been revised. Like earlier versions, the 2000 *Dietary Guidelines* (USDA/HHS, 2000) represent the basis for federal policy and are used to guide nutrition information, education, and interventions for federal, state, and local agencies. The guidelines, which are updated every 5 years, are based on current knowledge about how dietary intake may reduce the risk of major chronic diseases and how a healthful diet may promote health. They go well beyond the avoidance of dietary deficiencies; rather, they emphasize overall dietary patterns that can help to achieve favorable long-term health outcomes.

Although structured differently than the 1995 *Dietary Guidelines*, the 2000 *Dietary Guidelines* are similar in content, but include two new guidelines regarding food safety and physical activity (Box 1-6). Embedded in the guidelines is the Food Guide Pyramid—one of the major tools used for consumer nutrition education in the United States. The pyramid incorporates many of the *Dietary Guidelines* (see Chapter 4) and gives concrete recommendations that promote moderation, balance, and variety in food intake. Released in 1992, the pyramid reflects the 1989 Recommended Dietary Allowances for nutrients (NRC, 1989; USDA, 1992).

THE CHARGE TO THE COMMITTEE AND THE STUDY PROCESS

For the aforementioned reasons, FNS contracted with FNB to appoint a committee of experts to review the scientific basis for methods currently employed in the assessment of individuals for eligibility to the WIC program based on dietary risk. The committee's task was to evaluate the use of various dietary

> **BOX 1-6** The *Dietary Guidelines for Americans*
>
> AIM FOR FITNESS...
> - Aim for a healthy weight.
> - Be physically active each day.
>
> BUILD A HEALTHY BASE...
> - Let the Pyramid guide your food choices.
> - Choose a variety of grains daily, especially whole grains.
> - Choose a variety of fruits and vegetables daily.
> - Keep foods safe to eat.
>
> CHOOSE SENSIBLY...
> - Choose a diet that is low in saturated fat and cholesterol and moderate in total fat.
> - Choose beverages and foods to moderate your intake of sugars.
> - Choose and prepare foods with less salt.
> - If you drink alcoholic beverages, do so in moderation.
>
> SOURCE: USDA/HHS (2000).

assessment tools and to make recommendations for the assessment of inadequate or inappropriate dietary patterns. The focus of the evaluation was to be on tools that could accurately identify dietary risk of individuals and thus eligibility for participation in WIC. More specifically, the committee was charged with the following tasks:

- proposal of a framework for assessing dietary risk among WIC program applicants, focusing on *failure to meet Dietary Guidelines* as a risk criterion;
- identification and prioritization of areas of greatest concern when the *Dietary Guidelines* are incorporated into the WIC program;
- examination of the use of food-based and behavior-based approaches in assessing *failure to meet Dietary Guidelines* requirements specifically in the WIC setting;
- identification of specific cut-off points for any approaches identified as useful for establishing eligibility based on dietary risk; and
- identification of needed research and tools necessary for the implementation of any approaches identified as having the greatest potential for identifying those at nutrition risk.

Given that the *Dietary Guidelines* are not meant to be applied to children under the age of 2 years, the committee was requested to evaluate the above tasks only for women and for children over the age of 2 years.

In accordance with the IOM committee process, an expert committee was appointed with the above charge in mind. It was composed of nine individuals with a variety of professional degrees and with expertise in the areas of dietary assessment methodology, eating and behavior, dietetics, epidemiology, nutrition, obstetrics, public health, and pediatrics. A list of committee members, including a description of their backgrounds and expertise, is included in Appendix C.

The committee met five times over a 13-month period to consider its scope of work; review relevant evidence; and develop its findings, conclusions, and recommendations. To assist the committee in its deliberations, one meeting included a public workshop on Dietary Risk Assessment in the WIC Program on June 1, 2000, in Washington, D.C. Eight experts on various aspects of dietary assessment, four state WIC representatives whose states use different assessment methods and serve demographically diverse population groups, and two public policy experts gave formal presentations. During the workshop, interested individuals and organizations were invited to present both oral and written testimony to the committee. Overall, the workshop served to aid in the clarification of many important issues related to the committee's charge. The workshop agenda can be found in Appendix B.

Initially, the committee conducted a comprehensive search of the literature regarding dietary assessment methodology. All retrieved citations were reviewed to determine whether the citation was relevant to this report and, if relevant, whether to obtain the full paper. Throughout the study period, additional references were identified and obtained.

In December 1999, on behalf of IOM, NAWD regional directors requested all state agencies to send any currently used dietary assessment tools for the Committee on Dietary Risk Assessment's review. Characteristics of the tools submitted are reviewed in chapter 2. Committee members also visited local WIC clinics in their own geographic areas to familiarize themselves with current WIC clinic conditions and practices.

In September 2000, FNB/IOM released an interim report, *Framework for Dietary Risk Assessment in the WIC Program.* That report contained the framework for evaluating dietary risk assessment methods, summaries of presentations from the workshop on Dietary Risk Assessment, and the compilation of relevant citations from the literature.

ORGANIZATION OF THE REPORT

The report is organized into three sections:

- Chapters 1–3 set the stage for the report—giving an overview of the committee's statement of task and issues at hand, including a brief introduction to the WIC program and nutrition risk criteria, dietary risk and potential program benefits for eligible individuals, and the relationship of the *Dietary Guidelines* to the WIC population.

- Chapters 4–8 discuss the committee's framework for evaluating possible methods to assess dietary risk among WIC program applicants and review data bearing on the ability of food-based, physical activity-based, and behavioral-based assessment tools to classify individuals correctly on the basis of dietary risk.
- Chapter 9 presents a summary of the committee's findings and recommendations regarding the use of dietary, physical activity, and behavioral assessment tools in the WIC program.

2

Dietary Assessment Tools in WIC

Each state WIC agency uses its own standardized tools to collect dietary data. One of the committee's approaches was to review these tools to identify potential candidates for widespread use in eligibility determination related to *failure to meet Dietary Guidelines* or *inadequate diet*. Since dietary data collection tools are used for several purposes in WIC, this chapter briefly describes the uses that go beyond establishing dietary risk for eligibility purposes. It also summarizes the committee's findings about the types of tools that are in use for women and children, as well as the criteria that are applied in establishing eligibility.

PURPOSES OF DIETARY DATA COLLECTION

Dietary intake data are collected in WIC for three main purposes: (1) for determining dietary risk for eligibility purposes as discussed in Chapter 1, (2) as a starting place for nutrition education, and (3) for tailoring food packages. Because of the second and third uses, the dietary intake of a WIC applicant generally is assessed even if the applicant has already met eligibility requirements through other nutrition risk criteria. In fact, in 1998, 86 percent of state agencies had policies requiring that dietary information be obtained from all participants (Bartlett et al., 2000). Time constraints within the WIC program necessitate that the selected tools used provide information needed for all three uses.

Nutrition Education and Counseling

Federal regulations require nutrition education to be offered to each participant at least twice in each certification period (generally about 6 months). There are two broad goals of WIC nutrition education: (1) "to stress the relationship between proper nutrition and good health, with special emphasis on the nutritional needs of the program's target populations; and (2) to assist individuals at nutritional risk in achieving a positive change in food habits, resulting in improved nutritional status and the prevention of nutrition related problems" (Fox et al., 1998). The forms of education vary widely among agencies and types of participants. Frequently reported methods include individual counseling, group discussions, written materials, use of food models, food demonstrations, and video or slide show presentations (Bartlett et al., 2000). Education may be provided by a competent professional authority (CPA), who may be a professional or a paraprofessional staff member who has received basic training. Most education for high-risk individuals is provided by professional nutritionists. Nutrition education topics vary among types of participants and sites. Examples of commonly covered topics include the Food Guide Pyramid, diet for pregnancy, breastfeeding, and strategies to prevent or manage overweight.

An individual's self-described eating habits or patterns, in any form, can often be helpful to the CPA when choosing a starting place for nutrition education. Discussions of usual intake may help to establish rapport and also can uncover participant eating practices, disorders, or concerns to which WIC staff can respond appropriately with education or referral.

Food Package Tailoring

WIC participants receive supplemental food packages or instruments (vouchers or checks to be redeemed in retail grocery stores) in order to increase their intake of selected nutrients. Seven food packages are available for WIC participants: two for infants (age dependent); one for children 1–4 years of age; one for pregnant and breastfeeding women; one for postpartum, nonbreastfeeding women; an enhanced package for breastfeeding women; and specially tailored packages for women or children with special needs. The foods that make up the different packages are high in one or more nutrients that historically have been low in the diets of the program's low-income target population (i.e., protein, calcium, iron, and vitamins A and C). The foods provided include iron-fortified infant formula and infant and adult cereal, vitamin C-rich fruit and vegetable juices, eggs, milk, cheese, peanut butter, dried beans or peas, tuna fish, and carrots.

Approximately 98 percent of state WIC agencies adjust the contents of food packages to accommodate a participant's particular nutritional needs or preferences (Bartlett et al., 2000). Examples of the types of tailoring that are

TABLE 2-1 Nutritionally Related Food Package Tailoring Practices of WIC State Agencies

Tailoring Practice	Percent of State Agencies
Specific forms of formula are specified (ready-to-feed or powdered)	93
A specific form of food is specified for the convenience of the participant (powdered milk, juice concentrate)	82
Type of milk is specified (to reduce fat, lactose, or calories)	77
Amounts of certain food types are reduced (to meet age-related needs)	55
Amounts of certain food types are reduced (to reduce calories or nutrient intake for weight control)	49
Type of cheese is specified (to reduce fat)	28
Other methods (e.g., adjustment for food allergies)	25
Quantity of eggs is reduced (to reduce cholesterol)	19
Amounts of milk or juice are reduced	15
Type of cereal is specified (to reduce sucrose)	11

SOURCE: Bartlett et al. (2000).

made and the percentages of state agencies that practice each type of tailoring can be found in Table 2-1. The types of information useful for tailoring food packages include food allergies and intolerances, weight status, the availability of refrigeration or cooking appliances, and individual preferences within groups of nutrient-rich foods.

DIETARY ASSESSMENT TOOLS CURRENTLY USED BY WIC PROGRAMS

Most state and local WIC agencies may choose from more than one approved type of dietary assessment tool, depending on the circumstances. In 1998, 82 percent of states reported the use of 24-hour recalls and 80 percent reported the use of food frequency checklists (Bartlett et al., 2000). Other tools included dietary records (7 percent), computer-assisted analysis (8 percent), and other methods such as a diet history or questionnaires on feeding and eating practices (2 percent) (Bartlett et al., 2000).

In preparation for this study, the Nutrition Section of the National Association of WIC Directors asked each of the 88 state WIC agencies to submit current dietary assessment tools. A total of 54 agencies (43 states, 2 territories, and 9 Indian Tribal Organizations) responded to the request. Some agencies sent comprehensive explanations regarding the methods used to assess dietary risk; others sent only the tools being used. The tools varied in style from a blank box in which an individual could write her recollection of what was eaten the previous day to a four-page food frequency questionnaire that would allow a computer-generated summary of the dietary analysis.

State agencies used one of at least two different methods to categorize children: separate forms for infants and children ages 0–12 months, 12–24 months, and 2–5 years, or separate forms only for infants 0–12 months and children 1–5 years of age. Sixty-nine percent of the tools were designed to be self-administered, and 26 percent appeared to be interviewer-driven. The method of administration of the remaining 5 percent could not be determined. Although a few states used methods with a published research base, most used tools developed or adapted by state WIC agencies; they did not provide information about the validation of these tools. Although not specifically requested to submit the forms used for the ethnic groups served, many states did so, suggesting that many were attempting to meet the needs of their diverse populations.

Twenty-four-hour recalls capture a snapshot of an individual's diet over a 24-hour period. The procedures for obtaining 24-hour recalls can vary greatly. While a research-quality diet recall usually requires an interview of at least 20 minutes (Thompson and Byers, 1994; see Chapter 5), WIC time constraints generally preclude assessments of this length or intensity. The WIC tools used for collecting 24-hour recall data also vary considerably. For example, in Colorado, individuals are asked to write down everything eaten on a "typical" day. Other states (e.g., Florida) ask applicants to record all foods and beverages eaten the previous day and to mark an item indicating whether or not the day had been typical of eating habits. Staff in Arizona, using a similar recall method, then shade in the number of servings on a pyramid picture. Yet, in other states, recalls are interviewer-driven. Wyoming, among many states, stresses open-ended questions and the use of food models, measuring cups, and utensils to establish portion sizes typically consumed.

Food frequency questionnaires can vary greatly in design and number of food items, and those used by WIC vary greatly from state to state. Research-quality food frequency questionnaires that are intended to assess overall food or nutrient intake generally have 50 or more food items (see Chapter 5). Pennsylvania uses a 25-item questionnaire that categorizes foods into groups and obtains a daily number of servings from the five food groups of the Food Guide Pyramid (USDA, 1992, see Figure 2-1) by an unspecified method. Vermont uses a 39-item questionnaire and a simple arithmetic process to estimate the number of servings from the five Pyramid food groups. North Dakota uses an 84-item questionnaire and a simple computer program to produce a similar estimate. Some states use portion sizes in their questionnaires; others do not.

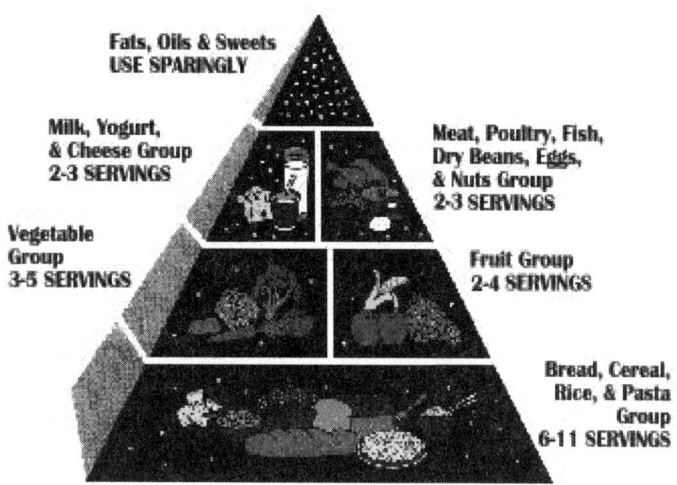

FIGURE 2-1 USDA Food Guide Pyramid.
SOURCE: USDA (1992).

In 1998, six state agencies reported using dietary records or food diaries (Bartlett et al., 2000). However, of states submitting assessment tools in 2000, including two states (North Carolina and West Virginia) that had reported using food records or diaries in 1998, none supplied tools that used this method.

As shown in Chapter 5, diet histories ordinarily obtain data such as usual meal patterns and food intake. The information about dietary assessment tools provided by the states to the U.S. Department of Agriculture suggests that a consistent definition of diet history is not used. In 1998, only one state, Indiana, reported using a diet history (Bartlett et al., 2000); but in 2000, nine states submitted tools labeled as "Diet History." Other tools labeled as "24-Hour Recall" actually appear to resemble modified diet histories. For example, several states used 24-hour recalls and then followed-up with questions regarding how typical the day had been and if not typical, what would be more typical? Some administered both a 24-hour recall and a short food-frequency questionnaire, which, when combined, are similar to a diet history. Depending on the participant responses and subsequent level of questioning, it can be difficult to classify assessment tools as one type or another.

Forty-six percent of states included some type of behavioral questions, but in most cases, it could not be determined whether the response would contribute in any way to the eligibility determination. Many tools included questions regarding physical activity, and some had questions to gain insight into food safety practices. A few forms also had questions that would indicate to staff whether the individual was at risk for food insecurity. States tended to use similar versions of the same tool for the different categories of participants.

An earlier examination of WIC dietary assessment tools included a checklist for dietary data collection instruments—primarily for food frequency questionnaires (Gardner et al., 1991). The committee noted that some of the WIC tools had many or most of the desirable characteristics identified in that list, but the list does not encompass all the key points presented in Chapter 4 of this report.

ELIGIBILITY CRITERIA IN USE

Review of the tools indicated that criteria used to establish dietary risk of women and children most often relate to the recommended numbers of servings from the Food Guide Pyramid. That is, the data obtained about food intake is converted to an estimated number of servings per day from the grains, fruit, vegetable, dairy, and meat and beans groups. (For more information about the Pyramid, see Chapter 3.) Few states provided information about the method used to assign combination or mixed foods to food groups.

Cut-off points to determine "at dietary risk" status vary greatly among the state WIC agencies. This variation occurs in the specification of the minimum number of servings from each food group and the number of deficiencies needed to establish dietary risk. For example, Arizona and Georgia use nine as the minimum number of servings from the grain group for pregnant women, whereas Illinois, Texas, and Delaware set the minimum number at six servings. In Arizona, if a participant falls short by only one serving in one food group, he or she qualifies as being at risk. In contrast, Texas not only requires deficiencies in three food groups before an individual qualifies as having an inadequate dietary pattern, but to make the criterion even more stringent, assigns only one deficiency if the person consumes at least some of the required servings from a food group.[1] For example, a pregnant women who consumes two out of the recommended six grain servings would be given a rating of only one deficiency. This woman would not have qualified based on the criterion for *inadequate diet* in Texas. Ironically, if this woman lived in Arizona, she would have been considered to be at dietary risk even if she had consumed an additional six servings (for a total of eight) from the bread group.

---

[1] Except for the fruits and vegetables food group. Within this food group, the lack of either a vitamin A-rich food or a vitamin C-rich food counts as a deficiency even if five fruits and vegetables are consumed.

SUMMARY

Tools for determining eligibility based on dietary risk also need to be useful for nutrition education and tailoring of the food package. Different WIC state agencies use many variations of 24-hour recalls and food frequency questionnaires. Similarly, the agencies use different criteria to identify dietary risk, but nearly all are based on the Food Guide Pyramid. After viewing the many variations of dietary assessment tools, it became apparent to the committee that the following needed review: the *Dietary Guidelines* and its embedded Food Guide Pyramid (Chapter 3), research on 24-hour recalls and food frequency questionnaires (Chapter 5), methods of physical activity assessment (Chapter 6), and approaches dealing with specific behaviors (Chapter 7).

3

Using the *Dietary Guidelines* as the Basis of Dietary Risk Criteria

The *Dietary Guidelines* are an integral part of WIC, just as they are of every federal program concerned with food, nutrition, or health. This chapter addresses the potential for using the *Dietary Guidelines* as the basis of one or more dietary risk criteria for establishing eligibility for WIC. It covers relationships among the *Dietary Guidelines*, WIC, and major goals of *Healthy People 2010* (HHS, 2000). Then it identifies the guidelines that the committee selected for special attention, advantages and disadvantages of *failure to meet Dietary Guidelines* as a risk criterion, and the rationale for the selection of guidelines for special attention.

THE *DIETARY GUIDELINES*, WIC, AND NATIONAL GOALS

The *Dietary Guidelines* are closely tied with the two major national goals presented in *Healthy People 2010* (HHS, 2000): (1) increase quality and years of healthy life, and (2) eliminate health disparities. Following the *Dietary Guidelines* helps Americans meet both those goals. The goal to eliminate health disparities is especially relevant to the WIC population. For nearly every nutrition objective covered in *Healthy People 2010*, groups that are heavily represented in WIC have baseline levels that are less favorable than the average. For example, 8 percent of low-income children ages 5 years and younger were growth retarded in 1997 (compared with an expected 5 percent) (HHS, 2000). Similarly, 12 percent of low-income children ($\leq$ 130 percent of poverty) ages 1 to 2 years had iron deficiency compared with 7 percent of children from families with incomes greater than 130 percent of poverty. Low-income people also are at increased risk for high levels of both morbidity and mortality associated with chronic diseases such as cardiovascular disease, diabetes, obesity, hypertension, and cancer (HHS, 2000).

WHICH *DIETARY GUIDELINES* SHOULD BE TARGETED?

A previous Institute of Medicine report recommended that *failure to meet Dietary Guidelines* be used as a criterion to establish dietary risk in WIC (IOM, 1996). Since a criterion consists of an indicator and a cut-off point, this means that the committee had to examine the *Dietary Guidelines* (USDA/HHS, 2000) for potential indicators and cut-off points. Recognizing that there are 10 guidelines, the committee addressed whether any of the 10 should be excluded from consideration—either because they are covered by other WIC nutritional risk criteria or because the guideline does not include a basis for setting a discrete, measurable cut-off point.

The WIC Policy Memorandum 98-9, Nutrition Risk Criteria (FNB, 1998; see Appendix A), which presents the nutrition risk criteria currently allowed in WIC, those not allowed, and those in need of further review, was examined. Although criterion number 401, *failure to meet Dietary Guidelines*, is an allowed criterion, it has not been standardized across WIC state agencies. Instead, a state WIC agency may base the criterion used on the definitions currently in use by that agency. (This situation relates to the need for the study by this committee.)

Summary of Guidelines Selected for Targeting

Table 3-1 lists each of the 10 guidelines in abbreviated form, the committee's decision regarding its relevance to the committee's work, and the reason, in brief, for that decision. Further details are provided in the text that follows.

Advantages and Disadvantages of Using the *Dietary Guidelines* to Establish Risk Criteria in WIC

The principal advantage of the *Dietary Guidelines* as a basis for dietary risk criteria is that the guidelines were developed for Americans from all backgrounds as a means to promote health. There are several obstacles to developing criteria for *failure to meet Dietary Guidelines*:

- The *Dietary Guidelines* are not intended for use for children under age 2 years; this restriction eliminates the use of the *Dietary Guidelines* for approximately 44 percent of the WIC population (USDA/HHS, 2000).

TABLE 3-1 Summary of the Committee's Decision to Review a Dietary Guideline Topic in Detail for Use in Setting Dietary Risk Criteria

Dietary Guideline Topic	Consider Further	Rationale
Healthy weight	No	Both underweight and overweight are already approved indicators of nutrition risk under the category of Anthropometric for all program applicants (see Appendix A). The *Dietary Guidelines* provide no indicators useful for identifying individuals at high risk of becoming overweight or underweight.
Physical activity	Yes	Strong relationship to weight and health, specific target activity levels are indicated (see Chapter 6).
Food Guide Pyramid	Yes	Specific target food group intakes are indicated for different energy levels. It is strongly related to at least two other guidelines (grains and fruits/vegetables) and also to the fat and sugars guidelines.
Grains	Yes[a]	Encompassed by the Pyramid guideline.
Fruits and vegetables	Yes[a]	Encompassed by the Pyramid guideline.
Food safety	No	Not readily operationalized into a criterion.
Saturated fat, fat, and cholesterol	Yes[a]	Covered in part by the Pyramid guideline.
Sugars	No	No quantitative recommendations.
Salt	No	A specific amount of salt is mentioned only indirectly and is the same for all individuals. Estimation of salt intake is very time-consuming.
Alcohol	No	Alcohol use is already an approved indicator of nutrition risk through the category of Clinical/Health/Medical (see Appendix A).

[a] Initially considered, but encompassed under the Food Guide Pyramid so not pursued individually.

- Some of the guidelines (i.e., Healthy Weight and Alcohol) already are covered by approved nutritional risk criteria (see Table 3-1).
- For the guidelines that do not have cut-off points specified, the committee has no basis for setting a cut-off point.

In the following sections, a brief discussion of each guideline and issues related to the development of a specific risk criterion for that guideline are presented.

Rationale for the Selection of Guidelines to Target

Aim for a Healthy Weight

Background. The focus of this guideline is on avoiding undesirable weight gain or losing weight gradually, if needed, in order to achieve a healthy weight. The purpose is to help people be fit and reduce their risk for high blood pressure, high blood cholesterol, heart disease, stroke, diabetes, certain types of cancer, arthritis, and breathing problems. Although not covered in the *Dietary Guidelines*, a healthy weight also promotes favorable reproductive outcomes (Galtier-Dereure et al., 1995, 2000). The guidance provided focuses on building a healthy base by eating vegetables, fruits, and grains with little added fat or sugar, selecting sensible portion sizes, and engaging in regular physical activity.

Issues Related to Setting a Dietary Risk Criterion. The *Dietary Guidelines* provide no clear basis for identifying intakes that are excessive or inadequate for maintaining a healthy weight. Since many elements are involved in achieving caloric balance, and since a small daily deficit or excess could lead to substantial weight change over time, it is not feasible to establish a practical and valid criterion concerning diet in relation to healthy weight.

Be Physically Active Each Day

Background. The specific physical activity recommendation in the *Dietary Guidelines* is to "aim to accumulate at least 30 minutes (adults) or 60 minutes (children) of moderate physical activity most days of the week, preferably daily." Moderate activity is defined, for adults, as "any activity that requires about as much energy as walking two miles in 30 minutes." Creating a separate guideline for physical activity was justified by the Dietary Guidelines Advisory Committee (2000) for the following reasons:

- the relationship between nutrition and physical activity goes beyond weight management;
- the health benefits of physical activity are extensive and intertwined with the health benefits of a healthful eating pattern;
- physical activity levels in the United States are lower than desirable; and
- people of all ages need to improve their physical activity levels regardless of their weight status.

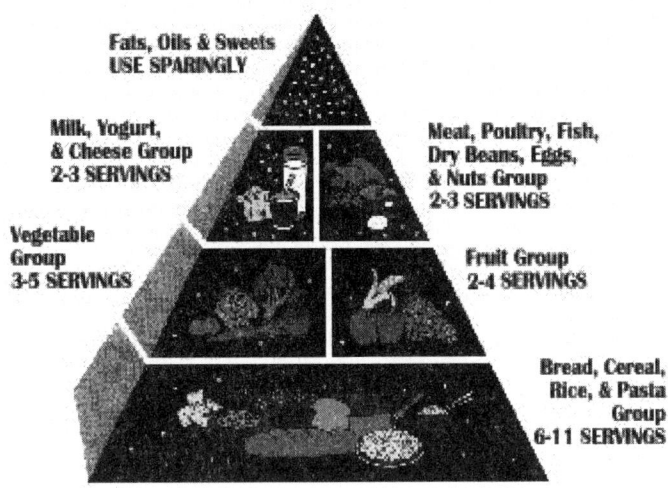

FIGURE 3-1 USDA Food Guide Pyramid.
SOURCE: USDA (1992).

Issues Related to Setting a Dietary Risk Criterion. As stated above, the guideline includes a minimum amount of activity that could be used to set a cut-off point for a criterion. Chapter 6 addresses this issue in detail.

Let the Pyramid Guide Your Food Choices

Background. *Let the Pyramid guide your food choices* replaces the guideline *Eat a variety of foods* from earlier editions of the *Dietary Guidelines* (Dietary Guidelines Advisory Committee, 2000). A major objective of the change was to use wording that would help ensure nutritional adequacy. The pyramid referred to in the guideline is the Food Guide Pyramid developed by the U.S. Department of Agriculture (USDA) (Figure 3-1). It provides concrete recommendations for the numbers of servings a person (ages 2 years or older) should consume from each of five basic food groups (grains, fruits, vegetables, milk products, and meat or beans) based on their energy needs (see Table 3-2). It also advises consumers to use fats, oils, and sweets sparingly. People who consume the recommended number of servings from each of the five basic groups in the Food Guide Pyramid are likely to have nutrient intakes that come close to the 1989 Recommended Dietary Allowances (NRC, 1989)—the intakes recommended at the time the Pyramid was developed (Cleveland, 1997)—rather

TABLE 3-2 Recommended Number of Pyramid Servings by Physiologic Status/Energy Intake and Food Group

Food Group	Children Ages 2–3 y (≈ 1,300 kcal)	Children Ages 4–6 y, Women (≈ 1,600 kcal)	Moderately Active Women, Some Pregnant Women (≈ 1,800 kcal)	Teen Girls; Active, Pregnant, or Lactating Women (≈ 2,200 kcal)
Grains group, especially whole grain	6	6	7	9
Vegetable group	3	3	3.3	4
Fruit group	2	2	2.3	3
Milk group, preferably fat free or low fat	2[a]	2 or 3[b]	2 or 3[b]	2 or 3[b]
Meat and beans group, preferably lean or low fat	2	2, for a total of 5 oz	2, for a total of 6 oz	2, for a total of 6 oz

[a] Portion sizes are reduced for children ages 2–3 years, except for milk.
[b] The number of servings from the milk group depends on age. Older children and teenagers (ages 9 to 18 years) need three servings daily. Women 19 years and older need two servings daily. During pregnancy and lactation, the recommended number of milk group servings is the same as for nonpregnant females of the same age.

SOURCE: Adapted from USDA/HHS (2000).

than the current Dietary Reference Intakes (DRIs) (IOM, 1997, 1998, 2000b, 2001).

From its inception, the Food Guide Pyramid was intended to be a dynamic nutrition education tool that is based on the *Dietary Guidelines* and nutrient recommendations, foods commonly consumed by Americans, and data on the nutrient content of those foods (Cronin, 1987). It was designed to allow consumers to choose foods they enjoy from each food group. In concept, the Pyramid incorporates the *Dietary Guidelines* and promotes good health, and it provides guidance for achieving nutrient adequacy without using supplements or highly fortified foods. Its design aims for balance and moderation along with nutrient adequacy. Notably, many state WIC agencies use the Food Guide

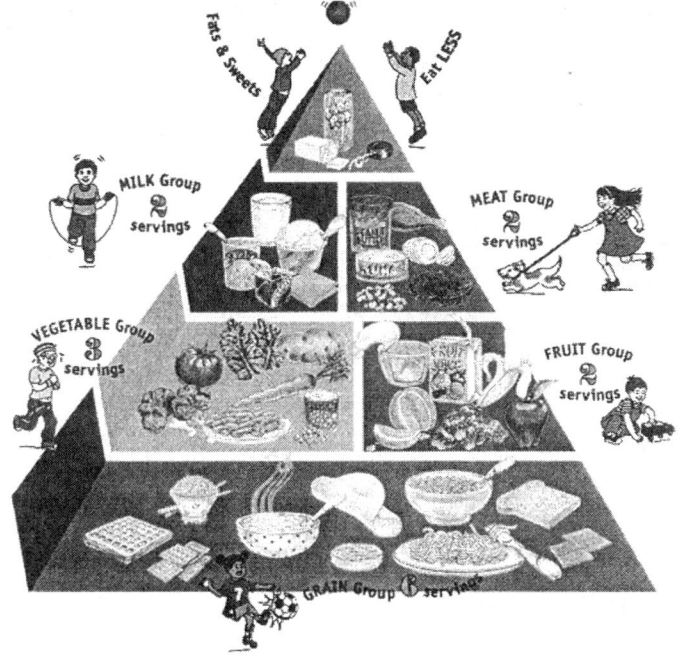

FIGURE 3-2 Children's Food Guide Pyramid.
SOURCE: Center for Nutrition Policy and Promotion (CNPP, 1999).

Pyramid to set specifications for the *failure to meet Dietary Guidelines* indicator.

The newer Children's Food Guide Pyramid, which is for children ages 2 to 6 years and their caregivers, has the same five food groups as the original Pyramid, but it lists only one recommended number of servings for each food group (the minimum number specified in Figure 3-2, which assumes an energy intake of 1,600 kcal/day) (Davis et al., 1999). The Children's Pyramid features nutritious foods commonly eaten by children and shows children engaged in active pursuits.

Issues Related to Setting a Dietary Risk Criterion. Is the Food Guide Pyramid a good tool to use to determine if a person is meeting the *Dietary Guidelines*? In some ways it is, but it is more complex than it appears. Based on the premise that the recommended numbers of servings for different energy levels are the numbers consistent with meeting the *Dietary Guidelines* and nutrient recommendations, the committee agreed that a cut-off point for each food group should be determined from Table 3-2. In other words, cut-off points for numbers of servings should be based on a person's estimated energy requirement and—for the milk group servings—a woman's age. For example, three servings of vegetables daily would be the cut-off point for a woman needing 1,600 kcal/day, but four servings would be the cut-off point for a woman needing 2,200 kcal/day. Two milk groups servings per day would be the cut-off point for a woman age 19 years or older, regardless of whether she was pregnant, lactating, or postpartum nonlactating. The challenge to WIC personnel is obtaining a reasonably accurate estimation of the person's energy requirement.

An advantage of using the Pyramid guidelines is that grains, vegetables, and fruits form the base of the Pyramid, and this is consistent with the emphasis on those foods in the next two guidelines listed below. The Food Guide Pyramid does less well, however, in addressing other parts of the *Dietary Guidelines*. It does not address physical activity or food safety (the two new guidelines) or alcohol at all. While the newer Food Guide Pyramid for Children (Davis et al., 1999) makes a small reference to physical activity through pictures of children engaged in activity, the original Food Guide Pyramid figure contains no clear guidance concerning how individuals should aim for a healthy weight. Although the accompanying educational materials do specify minimum numbers of servings to consume from the five recommended basic food groups for different energy levels, they do not provide maximum numbers. However, if excessive intake from one food group led to too few servings from another food group, the latter problem could be identified by comparison with the minimum. Neither the original nor the children's Pyramid provides a quantitative means to meet the other guidelines in the *choose sensibly* category—that is, guidelines for fat and cholesterol, sugars, and salt. Educational materials have been developed by USDA to support the Pyramid and provide this information, except for sugars (Shaw et al., 1996).

Using the Pyramid as a guide is intended to replace the need to evaluate one's diet on a nutrient-by-nutrient basis (Kennedy and Goldberg, 1995). Information is not available concerning how well the Pyramid provides for meeting revised recommended intake values that have been released in the DRI series (IOM, 1997, 1998, 2000b, 2001). Many of these new recommended intake values differ substantially from the ones used in developing the Pyramid before its release in 1992. The Pyramid has not been revised since its initial release—at least in part because the process of revising it would be complex and time-consuming (Shaw et al., 2000).

Despite its limitations, the committee considered *Let the Pyramid guide your food choices* promising as a practical and comprehensive guideline to use as a basis for determining if a person is at dietary risk because of *failure to meet Dietary Guidelines*. Consequently, it examined evidence related to the validity, reliability, and practicality of food-based questionnaires to assess whether an individual meets the *Dietary Guidelines* (see Chapter 5).

Eat a Variety of Grains Daily, Especially Whole Grains

Background. This guideline emphasizes whole grains because many of the health benefits of grains have been linked with whole grains rather than with refined grains. Components of whole grains may help reduce risk of chronic diseases such as coronary heart disease and certain types of cancer (Dietary Guidelines Advisory Committee, 2000). Whole grains also help promote normal bowel function. Both refined and whole grains provide the base of a healthful diet since many good-tasting choices are available that are low in fat, added sweeteners, and salt.

Issues Related to Setting a Dietary Risk Criterion. The text supporting this guideline is consistent with Food Guide Pyramid recommendations of at least six servings of grains per day (more for those with energy requirements greater than 1,600 kcal/day). The text also states "and include several servings of whole grain foods" and provides reasons for doing so, but it does not quantify the term "several." A risk criterion covering this guideline would fit under the guideline *Let the Pyramid guide your food choices*; however, it is unclear whether a cut-off should be set for whole grains.

Choose a Variety of Fruits and Vegetables Daily

Background. A generous intake of a variety of fruits and vegetables may help reduce the risk of chronic diseases such as heart disease and certain kinds of cancer. It also helps promote normal bowel function. Fruits and vegetables as a group tend to be good to excellent sources of many vitamins and minerals, as well as fiber. However, variety is important since a fruit rich in some vitamins and minerals may be low in others. Likewise, another fruit may have a different nutrient pattern altogether.

Issues Related to Setting a Dietary Risk Criterion. Again, the text supporting this guideline is consistent with Food Guide Pyramid recommendations: have a variety—including at least two servings of fruits and three servings of vegetables daily. It is unclear whether or how to translate "choose a variety" into a dietary risk criterion. The text advises consumers to choose dark-green leafy vegetables, orange fruits and vegetables, and cooked dry beans and peas often, but it does not specify frequency. Risk criteria covering the fruits and vegetable guideline would fit under the guideline *Let the Pyramid guide your food choices*.

Keep Food Safe to Eat

Background. Food safety is relevant to WIC's target population because pregnant women, infants, and young children are at high risk for food-borne illness and the consequences of food-borne illness may be serious—even life-threatening. Risk is especially high for people with weakened immune systems, such as mothers or infants who are infected with human immunodeficiency virus, many of whom are served by WIC.

Healthful eating depends on consuming food that is safe from harmful bacteria, viruses, parasites, and chemical contaminants. Although farmers, food producers, and food handlers in markets and eating establishments all play important roles in keeping food safe to eat, women and caregivers can take concrete steps to protect themselves and the infants and children in their care.

Issues Related to Setting a Dietary Risk Criterion. Criteria pertaining to this guideline would need to focus on one or more of the seven subguidelines in the *Dietary Guidelines*:

- Clean. Wash hands and surfaces often.
- Separate. Separate raw, cooked, and ready-to-eat foods while shopping, preparing, or storing.
- Cook. Cook foods to a safe temperature.
- Chill. Refrigerate perishable foods promptly.
- Check and follow the label.
- Serve safely. Keep hot foods hot and cold foods cold.
- When in doubt, throw it out.

The supporting text in the *Dietary Guidelines* provides specifics that could be used to set numerous criteria, for example, criteria concerning handwashing, safe temperatures, and maximum times for holding foods at temperatures in the danger zone. However, operationalizing these behaviors for the purpose of determining WIC eligibility would be difficult. The guideline does not lend itself to a criterion-based reference. Moreover, the committee found no tested questionnaires or related research to use as a basis for considering food safety as an indicator of practices in the criterion category *failure to meet Dietary Guidelines*. Therefore, the committee discontinued consideration of this dietary guideline for setting a dietary risk criterion.

Choose a Diet that is Low in Saturated Fat and Cholesterol and Moderate in Total Fat

Background. Strong evidence indicates that high intakes of saturated fat and cholesterol contribute to the development of coronary heart disease. The contribution of fat to obesity and to other chronic diseases is less certain. Compared with earlier editions of the *Dietary Guidelines*, the latest edition places greater emphasis on lowering saturated fat intake. The text provides suggestions for doing this, covering sources of saturated fats and possible alternatives. The text places less emphasis on restricting total fat intake.

Issues Related to Setting a Dietary Risk Criterion. The *Dietary Guidelines* specifies "no more than 30 percent of calories from total fat" and "less than 10 percent of calories from saturated fat" should be consumed in one day. Both the *Dietary Guidelines* and the Food Guide Pyramid specify an upper limit on total fat intake as a percentage of food energy for the day and suggest about 300 mg of cholesterol as a maximum average daily intake. However, only the *Dietary Guidelines* presents reasons why the percentage of energy from total fat should not be much below 30 percent. When the fruit or grain recommendation is not met, the percentage of energy from fat may become excessive (Krebs-Smith et al., 1997). The Pyramid guideline would only partially cover the fat guideline.

Choose Beverages and Foods to Moderate Your Intake of Sugars

Background. The guideline to moderate intake of sugars is intended to reduce risk of tooth decay and help avoid excess calories. The focus is on added sweeteners, not the sugars that occur naturally in fruit and milk products.

Issues Related to Setting a Dietary Risk Criterion. The text accompanying the guideline provides no specific guidance regarding what quantity of sweeteners would be excessive. Rather, it encourages consumers to get most of their calories from grains, fruits, vegetables, low-fat or non-fat dairy products, and lean meats or meat substitutes. It warns against letting soft drinks or other sweets crowd out more nutritious foods. The *Dietary Guidelines* provide no quantitative basis for setting a dietary risk criterion based on intake of sweeteners. Consequently, the committee did not consider this guideline further in relation to setting dietary risk criteria.

Choose and Prepare Foods with Less Salt

Background. The principal intent of this guideline is reduction of the risk of hypertension (high blood pressure). The rate of hypertension is greater in low-income populations (32 percent) than in middle- or high-income populations (27 percent), and is greater in African-American individuals (40 percent) than in white individuals (27 percent) (HHS, 2000). Based on data from the 1988–1991 National Health and Nutrition Examination Survey, 39 to 68 percent of U.S. women ages 50 to 79 years have hypertension, as do 48 to 73 percent of African-American women (HHS, 2000).

Issues Related to Setting a Dietary Risk Criterion. The guideline does not state a specific cut-off point for salt or sodium. Rather, it refers to the Daily

Value of 2,400 mg of sodium specified on Nutrition Facts Labels and mentions that the need for sodium is actually much less. A majority of the salt in U.S. diets comes from salt added during food processing or during preparation in a food establishment or at home. Thus, estimating the amount of salt provided by the foods consumed would require detailed information from food labels and from people involved in food preparation—along with information about the consumer's addition of salt and salty seasonings. For these several reasons, the committee did not consider this guideline further for setting dietary risk criteria.

If You Drink Alcoholic Beverages, Do So in Moderation

Background. The text of *Dietary Guidelines* points out many adverse effects of excess alcohol intake and makes it clear that women under age 55 years are unlikely to benefit from alcohol consumption. It names groups that should not drink alcoholic beverages at all, including children, adolescents, and women who may become pregnant or who are pregnant. The concern for women who may become pregnant relates to the high rate of unplanned pregnancies in the United States and the risk of birth defects from alcohol consumption even in the first few weeks of pregnancy (Dietary Guidelines Advisory Committee, 2000). Breastfeeding women (especially those not breastfeeding exclusively) are among the women who may become pregnant.

Issues Related to Setting a Dietary Risk Criterion. The approved medical risk criterion for alcohol intake by pregnant women (see Appendix A) is compatible with the *Dietary Guidelines*—that is, a cut-off point of any alcohol use. The approved medical risk criterion concerning alcohol intake by breastfeeding women is much more lenient than a criterion that would be derived from the *Dietary Guidelines* (i.e., a cut-off point of any alcohol use), but medical risk places the approved criterion in Priority I—a much higher priority than is given to dietary risk. Consequently, the committee gave no further consideration to the use of alcohol as a dietary risk criterion.

Summary

The most promising approach to using the *Dietary Guidelines* for establishing dietary risk criteria for the WIC program is to focus on the single guideline *Let the Pyramid guide your food choices*. The major advantages and disadvantages are summarized in Box 3-1.

BOX 3-1 Major Advantages and Disadvantages of Focusing on *Let the Pyramid Guide Your Food Choices* to Evaluate Dietary Risk Based on *Failure to meet Dietary Guidelines*

Advantages
- Following the guideline, *Let the Pyramid guide your food choices*, helps ensure nutrient adequacy according to the 1989 Recommended Dietary Allowances (NRC, 1989).
- The Pyramid guideline covers at least two other guidelines: *Eat a variety of grains daily . . .* and *Choose a variety of fruits and vegetables daily*.
- Meeting recommendations for grains, fruits, and vegetables also may reflect moderation in intake of fats and sugars.
- The guideline provides a basis for definite cut-off points for each of the five basic food groups based on energy needs.

Disadvantages
- The Food Guide Pyramid has not been updated to reflect new nutrient recommendations reflected in the Dietary Reference Intakes (IOM, 1997, 1998, 2000b, 2001).
- The Pyramid does not address physical activity or any aspect of food safety or salt intake.
- Energy needs are difficult to estimate accurately, and these affect the recommended servings of food groups.
- The Pyramid guideline provides no practical way to set cut-off points that relate to dietary aspects of aiming for a healthy weight or limiting intakes of saturated fat and sugars.
- The physical activity guideline merits further examination.

4

Framework for Evaluating Tools to Assess Dietary Risk

During early deliberations, the Committee on Dietary Risk Assessment in the WIC Program developed a framework for evaluating methods to assess dietary risk in WIC program applicants. The committee's overall goal was to identify an assessment tool that could determine whether individuals did or did not meet the *Dietary Guidelines for Americans* (USDA/HHS, 2000) or more specifically (as discussed in Chapter 3) *Let the Pyramid guide your food choices*. It also considered the potential of tools to identify nutrient intakes in relation to cut-off points since diet adequacy is another allowed type of criterion (see Appendix A). This chapter outlines eight characteristics that together provide a framework for evaluating the usefulness and effectiveness of a dietary risk assessment tool in the WIC setting. Based on further deliberations, this framework has been modified slightly from that presented in the committee's interim report (IOM, 2000c).

DESIRABLE CHARACTERISTICS OF AN ASSESSMENT TOOL

1. The Tools Should Identify Dietary Risks that are Related to Health or Disease

Ideally, any risk criterion adopted for dietary risk should be both predictive of the individual's risk of health problems as well as indicative of nutrition and health benefit from program participation. When considering health outcomes for children, appropriate growth and development are key facets of health. Diet has been shown to have both short- and long-term effects on behavior, cognitive development, physical growth, and general health status (Levitsky and Strupp, 1995; Pollitt, 1988). Inadequate energy intake in early life may be directly linked to poor outcomes in cognitive function, such as learning, or nutritional status in childhood (Gorman, 1995). Infants, preschool, and school-age children who are iron-deficient show deficits in mental development, attention, and learning, as well as in achievement test scores, when compared to iron-replete children (CDC, 1998b). In addition, essential fatty acids are necessary for proper brain development (Uauy et al., 2000).

For children ages 2 to 5 years and pregnant or postpartum women, the 1996 IOM WIC report suggested using the indicator *failure to meet Dietary Guidelines* (IOM, 1996). As discussed in Chapter 3, this would involve using the updated consensus document, *Dietary Guidelines for Americans* (USDA/HHS, 2000), as a reference, specifically as related to the two guidelines, *Let the Pyramid guide your food choices* and *Be physically active each day*.

In screening situations, one is assessing how an individual's dietary intake compares with an appropriate cut-off point based on the *Dietary Guidelines*. The purpose is to conclude whether the individual "meets" or "does not meet" the *Dietary Guidelines*. For such vulnerable populations as pregnant women, postpartum women, and children ages 2 to 5 years, the committee decided that many criteria could be set, any one of which would provide evidence that the individual fails to meet either the Food Pyramid guideline or the physical activity guideline (see Chapters 3, 5, and 6).

2. The Tools are Appropriate for Age and Physiological Condition

Several subgroups are served in the WIC program: pregnant, breastfeeding, and nonbreastfeeding women, along with their infants and children younger than 5 years of age. When assessing dietary risk, consideration needs to be given to the specific nutritional recommendations and appropriate dietary patterns for these groups. For example, if a tool were to assess whether a client consumes the recommended number of servings of fruits and vegetables, it would need to be designed to accommodate different recommendations for adult women as compared to young children and differences in common food choices by these two groups. A second consideration relates to the method of administration of the tool for assessing dietary risk. For example, young children cannot report their dietary intake, and proxy (parental) reports must be used. Hence, one must evaluate the suitability of tools for each client subgroup.

3. The Tools Should Ideally Serve Three Purposes: Screening for Eligibility, Individualizing the Food Package, and Nutrition Education for Behavior Change

As discussed in Chapter 2, dietary assessment tools are utilized for three reasons in the WIC setting: to define dietary risk as a criterion for eligibility in the WIC program, to identify eating patterns that influence the type of supplemental food package provided by the program, and as the starting point for nutrition education and counseling efforts. Ideally, one tool could be used for these purposes; however, the committee recognized that the standards for the effectiveness of a tool for screening would likely be higher than those required if the tool is used primarily for education. In the latter case, less well-performing tools would still have utility for education purposes if they provided the WIC nutrition professional with sufficient background on the individual's food choices from which to begin a dialogue regarding dietary change.

4. The Tools Should have Acceptable Performance Characteristics

All instruments should be evaluated prior to use to ensure that they perform adequately. Performance is assessed in quantitative terms by considering the validity and reliability of the instrument (Windsor et al., 1994), and related constructs that are defined in Table 4-1. Validity addresses whether one is really measuring what was intended. For example, 24-hour dietary recalls are intended to measure dietary intake for the previous 24-hour period, but several recent studies have revealed that as much as 30 percent of foods reported by children were not eaten the previous day (Baxter et al., 1997). Foods reported but not eaten are called intrusions or phantom foods (Domel et al., 1994). A method that systematically under- or overestimates consumption leads to biased estimates and is therefore not considered valid. Reliability relates to whether applying the same instrument two or more times provides the same results (Table 4-1). Reliability thereby indicates the degree of random error in the dietary assessment method. Random error could be caused by such conditions as the respondent or interviewer being upset at the time of assessment, multiple interviewers, excessive noise during assessment, the limitations of memory, or a person's inability to properly average intake to provide a desired response on a food frequency questionnaire. Random error is always present; therefore, the question when evaluating a tool is whether the level of random error present is acceptable for the intended purpose. Chapter 5 provides further information about error in dietary data collection and the performance of different types of data collection tools used to assess diet.

Error in the assessment of the dietary intake of an individual leads to misclassification in the determination of eligibility for the WIC program. Misclassification has serious consequences in that some truly eligible individuals

TABLE 4-1 Terms Used When Describing or Evaluating the Performance Characteristics of an Assessment Tool

Term	Definitions
Validity	Does the method measure what it is supposed to measure?
	Is the method accurate? That is, does it provide an unbiased estimate of usual dietary intake?
Bias	Also known as systematic error
	If biased, the estimated mean intake is not equal to the true mean intake
Reliability	Refers to the ability of the estimate to be reproduced when the measure is repeated
	The inability of the measure to be reproduced is a function of the amount of random error in the assessment procedure
Reproducibility	See Reliability
Random error	Variability in the measure when assessed over time
	Increases the variance around the mean of the measure, but does not affect the estimate of the mean
	Random error is inversely related to reliability
Between-individual variability	Variability across individuals in their usual dietary intakes
	Considered the true variability when estimating intakes of groups
Within-individual variability	Variability in dietary intakes within an individual from day to day
	Reduces the reliability of the measurement of usual intake
Measurement error or imprecision	Refers to error in dietary intake estimation due to the measurement process itself
	Includes interviewer differences, food composition database errors
	Reduces the reliability and validity of the measurement of usual intake
Misclassification	Quantification of error within the context of classifying individuals as being at dietary risk
	Quantified in terms of Sensitivity and Specificity of the measure
Sensitivity	Refers to the proportion or percent of individuals with dietary risk who are identified by the assessment tool as being at dietary risk
Specificity	Refers to the proportion or percent of individuals not at dietary risk who are identified by the assessment tool as not being at dietary risk
Positive predictive value	Refers to the proportion or percent of individuals identified at dietary risk who are truly at dietary risk
Negative predictive value	Refers to the proportion of individuals identified to not be at dietary risk who are truly not at dietary risk

may not be classified as eligible for the services (less than perfect sensitivity), or individuals not truly eligible for the services may receive them (less than perfect specificity). Chapter 5 provides examples of the effects of less than perfect sensitivity and specificity. In the absence of perfect tools (tools with 100 percent sensitivity and 100 percent specificity), policymakers and the public must decide how much and what type of misclassification error they are willing to tolerate when certifying people to receive or not receive federally funded WIC services. It is the view of the committee that less than perfect specificity should be tolerated in order to achieve perfect sensitivity; in other words, to ensure that all truly eligible individuals are identified as eligible with existing assessment tools, it is acceptable that some truly noneligible individuals receive WIC services.

5. The Tools Should be Suitable for the Culture and Language of the Population Served

The WIC program serves a multiethnic, multicultural, heterogeneous population. Thirty-nine percent of WIC participants are Caucasian, 33 percent are Latino, 23 percent are African American, 3 percent are Asian or Pacific Islander, and 2 percent are American Indian or Alaskan Native (Bartlett et al., 2000). The percentages of non-Caucasians and the diversity of cultures are expected to increase. Diversity in heritage, geography, food consumed, and culture translates into diversity in dietary patterns and practices. To assess dietary intake and patterns effectively, dietary assessment tools would need to be developed with each specific culture in mind. Thus, many WIC agencies would require several dietary assessment tools to serve their population mix. Language translation alone would not provide an acceptable tool for a different culture because the types of foods consumed, the portion sizes, food combinations, and the way foods and eating are conceptualized are likely to differ.

It is true that standardized 24-hour recalls and food records capture cultural preferences and foods consumed, provided that the interviewer is knowledgeable about reported foods, follows standard methods, and uses a food composition database that includes the foods. Thus, the need to consider specific development of tools for different cultural groups refers to the use of food frequency methods to determine usual dietary intakes. It was also recognized that effective administration of tools to different cultural groups would likely require special training and that little information exists to document successful adaptations of dietary assessment instruments for use in different cultures whose members wish to use WIC services.

6. The Tools Should be Responsive to Operational Constraints in the WIC Setting

Time constraints for both staff and participants necessitate the use of an assessment tool that can be administered, scored, and interpreted rapidly. It is imperative that the tools under consideration take into account the variety of skills and knowledge levels of the competent professional authorities (CPAs) who assess dietary intake in the WIC setting. Whether CPAs are paraprofessional or professional, the assessment and educational tools they use need to be linguistically and culturally appropriate for different population groups served by WIC clinics.

A tool should provide consistent results regardless of the staff member who administers it. Subjective measures in scoring should be avoided to eliminate administrator bias. Furthermore, the tool should be constructed in a manner so as not to influence the client. Features that may influence responses inappropriately include scoring mechanisms placed directly on a self-administered form and phrasing that invites desirable or favorable responses rather than accurate ones. Additional points that need to be considered include the impact of the tools on the systems used by the WIC agency, and expected future changes to the system, such as automation or computerization.

7. The Tools Should be Standardized Across States and Agencies

To some degree, tools used to determine eligibility for WIC participation based on dietary risk need to be standardized across state agencies for each of the categorical groups served by WIC. While differences in culture and language preclude the use of a single tool in all settings or even in a single setting, some form of standardization needs to occur to ensure equal access to program benefits regardless of the individual's place of residence or cultural background. Moreover, if federal funding for the program is limited, standardization could help to ensure that individuals at greatest risk and with potential to benefit are served first.

Standardization of dietary assessment tools and their interpretation can also facilitate tracking program benefits and comparing program activities and results across states. Program efficiencies may be gained by the broader use of standardized tools. These efforts could provide a stronger information base for the U.S. Department of Agriculture (USDA) and states to track program operations and uses of dietary risk assessment in WIC. For example, a few years ago, states were interested in having a common tool to assess the risk of food insecurity/hunger. USDA has since developed a food security module (USDA, 2001a) which, if used by states collecting this type of data, will allow comparison to data on a national level.

8. The Tools Should Allow for Prioritization Within the Category of Dietary Risk

Currently, funding for the supplemental food assistance portion of WIC is sufficient to meet current participation levels, and all who apply and meet eligibility criteria receive the food assistance component of WIC. However, if and when resources for WIC are insufficient to serve all those eligible, a tool should allow the prioritization of risk within the dietary risk category. The goal should be to ensure that those at greatest dietary risk and those most likely to benefit are served first. Meeting this goal requires a set of criteria that has different degrees of stringency reflecting different degrees of risk.

SUMMARY

These eight criteria formed the framework used by the committee for evaluating tools to assess dietary risk. In order to be a desirable tool, it must:

- use specific criteria that are related to health or disease;
- be appropriate for age and physiological condition;
- serve three purposes: screening for eligibility, tailoring of food packages, and nutrition education;
- have acceptable performance characteristics (validity and reliability);
- be suitable for the culture and language of the population served;
- be responsive to operational constraints in the WIC setting;
- be standardized across states and agencies; and
- allow prioritization within the category of dietary risk.

5

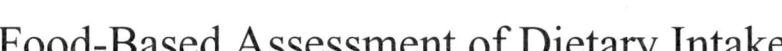

Food-Based Assessment of Dietary Intake

This chapter addresses the question, What food-based dietary assessment methods hold promise for eligibility determination in WIC based on criteria related to either *failure to meet Dietary Guidelines* (indicated primarily by not meeting Food Guide Pyramid recommendations) or *inadequate intake* (indicated by falling below nutrient intake cut-off points based on Dietary Reference Intakes)? To answer the question, the committee examined the scientific basis for the potential performance of food-based methods for eligibility determination at the individual level. This examination required consideration of relevant dietary research at the group level. The committee was most interested in reviewing studies of dietary methods designed to assess the usual[1] or long-term intakes of individuals and groups, especially those methods that may have the characteristics that meet the criteria for assessing dietary risk described in Chapter 4. To the extent possible, the committee focused on studies conducted with populations served by WIC: women in the childbearing years, children younger than 5 years of age, and low-income women and children from diverse ethnic backgrounds.

The term *food-based dietary assessment methods* refers to assessment tools used to estimate the usual nutrient or food intake of an individual or a group. Dietary intake is self-reported by individuals (since direct observation of intake by trained observers is impractical), and therefore poses greater challenges than does using anthropometric or biochemical measures for the determination of

---

[1] Usual intake is defined as the long-run average intake of food, nutrients, or a specific nutrient for an individual (IOM, 2000a).

WIC eligibility. To use a dietary method to assess an individual's dietary risk of *failure to meet Dietary Guidelines* or *inadequate intake*, the method must have acceptable performance characteristics (described in Chapter 4). The committee focused on available dietary tools with regard to their ability to estimate usual intake and their performance characteristics (validity, reliability, measurement error, bias, and misclassification error). The intent was to determine how well the tools could identify an individual's WIC eligibility status based on the dietary risk of *failure to meet Dietary Guidelines* or *inadequate intake*. The committee considered data related to the correct identification of intakes of nutrients, foods, and food groups since elements from any of these three groupings could be used as the indicator on which a criterion could be based. For example, a method to identify *failure to meet Dietary Guidelines* must be able to identify accurately a person's usual intake from each of the five basic food groups of the Food Guide Pyramid.

This chapter describes (1) the importance of assessing *usual* intake, (2) commonly used research-quality dietary assessment methods, including their strengths and limitations, (3) methods that compare food intakes with the *Dietary Guidelines*, and (4) conclusions about food-based methods for eligibility determination.

A FOCUS ON USUAL INTAKE

As explained below, dietary assessment for the purpose of determining WIC eligibility must be based on long-term intake or the usual pattern of dietary intake, rather than intake reported for a single day or a few days. In the United States and other developed countries, a person's dietary intake varies substantially from day to day (Basiotis et al., 1987; Carriquiry, 1999; IOM, 2000a; Nelson et al., 1989; Tarasuk, 1996; Tarasuk and Beaton, 1999). This variation introduces random error in estimates of usual intake. Day-to-day variation in intake arises from multiple biologic and environmental influences such as appetite, physical activity, illness, season of the year, holidays, and personal economic conditions. An individual's intake may become either more erratic or more monotonous when economic constraints are added to other influences on dietary intake.

Relationships Among Daily Nutrient Intakes, Usual Intakes, and a Cut-Off Point

Figure 5-1 presents distributions of intake for a hypothetical nutrient X that is normally distributed. It depicts the relationship between the distributions of usual intakes of individuals within a population and the distribution of usual intake for that population (solid line P). L marks the cut-off point for determining whether an individual's usual intake is above or below a specified cut-off

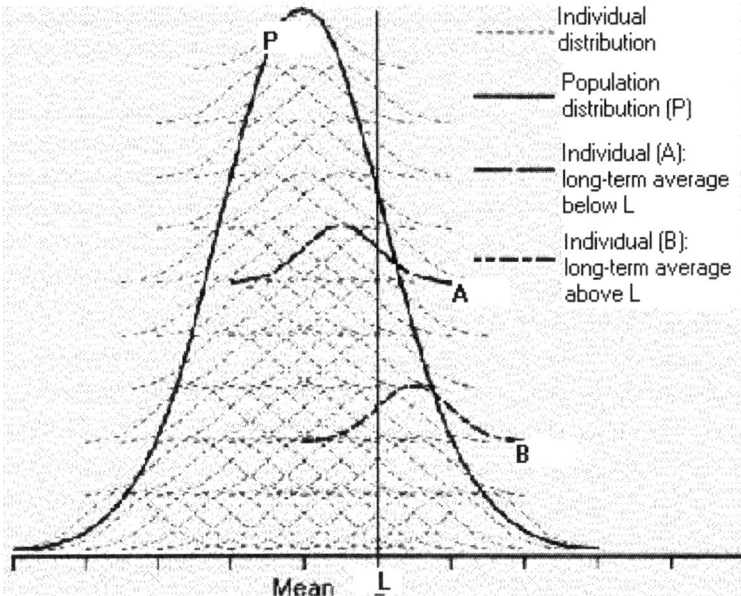

FIGURE 5-1 Relationship Between Distributions of Usual Intakes of Nutrient X for Individuals Within a Population (P) and a Generic Cut-Off Level L.
SOURCE: Adapted from Yudkin (1996).

level L. The individual values reflected in a dotted line represent the day-to-day intakes of an individual that taken together comprise usual intake. On any given day, Individual A and Individual B can have a dietary intake for a specified nutrient that is at, above, or below L. However, Individual A has a long-term average intake (usual intake) below cutpoint L, whereas Individual B has an average or usual intake above cutpoint L. Compared with a set of recalls, a single recall or day of observation would identify many more individuals as falling below L for most nutrients. Therefore, the accurate approximation of an individual's usual intake requires data collection over many days (Basiotis et al., 1987; Beaton, 1994; IOM, 2000a; Sempos et al., 1993).

Identifying Who Falls Above or Below a Cut-Off Point

Estimating the proportion of a population *group* with a nutrient intake above or below L requires the collection of one day of intake data per person in the population plus an independent second day of intake for at least a subsample of the population (Carriquiry, 1999; IOM, 2000a; Nusser et al., 1996). This procedure allows for statistical adjustment of the distribution of nutrient intake for the group. That is, with data from 2 days, one can account for the day-to-day variation in intake that is described in the previous section. The statistical methods used account for day-to-day variability of intake in the population and other factors such as day-of-the-week and the skewness of the intake of nutrient X. However, no method based on one or two recalls is available to identify whether an *individual's* usual intake would be above or below L.

Variability in Food Intake

Turning from nutrients to foods, some individuals are relatively consistent in their intake of a few foods (such as low-fat milk or coffee) from day to day, but they may vary widely in their intake of other foods (e.g., corn or watermelon) (Feskanich et al., 1993). Available data suggest that within-person variability is at least as great a problem in estimating an individual's *food* intake as it is in estimating an individual's *nutrient* intake. In a German study based on 12 diet recalls per person collected over 1 year, the ratio of within-person to between-person variation in food group consumption was greater than 1.0 for nearly all of the 24 food groups included (Bohlscheid-Thomas et al., 1997). The ratio of within-person to between-person variation ranged from 0.6 for spreads to 65.1 for legumes. The high ratios[2] reflect large day-to-day within-person variation in the consumption of different foods.

In summary, a large body of literature indicates that day-to-day variation in nutrient and food intake is so large in the United States that one or two diet recalls or food records cannot provide accurate information on usual nutrient and food intake for an individual.

OVERVIEW OF RESEARCH-QUALITY DIETARY METHODS FOR ESTIMATING FOOD OR NUTRIENT INTAKE

A large body of literature addresses the performance of methods developed to assess dietary intakes and conduct research on diet and health. Four methods—diet history, diet recall (typically 24-hours), food record, and food frequency questionnaire (FFQ)—have been widely studied (Bingham, 1987; Dwyer, 1999; IOM, 2000a; Pao and Cypel, 1996; Tarasuk, 1996; Thompson and Byers, 1994). Most studies of dietary data collection methods focus on the ability of a method to estimate nutrient intake accurately—ranging from just one nutrient to a wide array of them. Some studies examine performance with re-

---

[2] The within-person variability is an individual's day-to-day variability in reported intakes (or intraindividual variability or standard deviation within). The between-person variability (or interindividual variability) is the variability in intakes from person to person. A higher ratio of within- to between-person variability means that the variability of the food or nutrient intake is greater within an individual than the variability between individuals.

spect to intake of foods or food groups. The findings discussed in this chapter highlight 24-hour diet recalls and food frequencies, since these are the most commonly used dietary methods in the WIC clinic (see Chapter 2).[3]

General Characteristics

The strengths and limitations of available dietary methods have been extensively reviewed elsewhere (Bingham, 1987; Briefel et al., 1992; Dwyer, 1999; Pao and Cypel, 1996; Tarasuk, 1996; Willett, 2000) and are summarized in Table 5-1. Each of the four methods may be used to provide nutrient intake data, food intake data, or both. Table 5-1 also presents major findings that have implications for use of each of the four methods in the WIC program. In addition, after providing descriptive information about the methods, the table presents two major groups of characteristics that are related to the framework described in Chapter 4—performance characteristics and characteristics related to responsiveness to operational constraints in the WIC setting. These characteristics include the resources required to administer the method (WIC staff, time, and facilities such as computer software), and burden and ability of the client to report or record intake accurately.

As shown in Table 5-1, the diet history and FFQ methods attempt to estimate the usual intake of individuals over a long period of time, often the past year. The 24-hour diet recall and food record methods reflect intake over 1 day or a few days. As discussed in the previous section, recalls and records are not good measures of an individual's usual intake unless a number of independent days are observed.[4] On average, diet recalls and food records tend to underestimate usual intake—energy intake in particular. On the other hand, FFQs and diet histories tend to overestimate mean energy intakes, depending on the length of the food lists that are used and subjects' abilities to estimate accurately the frequency and typical portion sizes of foods they consume.

Methods Studies Conducted with Low-Income Women and Children

Table 5-2 summarizes the few dietary methods studies that have been conducted with low-income pregnant women and young children or in the WIC population. These studies have been primarily aimed at developing or testing the

---

[3] The dietary history method used in the WIC clinic is not necessarily the traditional diet history method, which takes about one to two hours to administer properly. Food records are not often used because of time limitations and difficulties obtaining complete and accurate records.

[4] For some nutrients (such as vitamin A) that are highly concentrated in certain foods, or foods that are eaten sporadically, many days or months of intake may be needed to accurately estimate the usual intake of an individual (IOM, 2000a).

TABLE 5-1 Comparison of Performance and Operational Constraints of Selected Dietary Assessment Methods in the WIC Setting

Criterion or Characteristic	Diet History	24-Hour Diet Recall
Definition of diet method	An interviewer conducts a 1–2 hr interview with a respondent (or proxy for a child) to ask usual meal patterns, food intake, and other information related to diet Typically includes two or more diet methods (food frequency questionnaire [FFQ], 24-hr diet recall, 3-d food record, or questionnaire on dict behaviors), but a standardized method is not available	An interviewer asks the respondent (or proxy for a child) to recall all foods and beverages consumed yesterday (for a 24-hr period such as midnight to midnight); food descriptions and amounts for each food are recalled; amounts are estimated using portion size measurement aids
Ability to estimate usual food or nutrient intake (an individual's average intake over a long period of time)	Yields a more representative pattern of usual intakes in the past than other methods; generally designed to assess total diet Tends to overestimate nutrient intakes compared with diet recall and food record Provides information on the frequency and types of foods typically eaten, preparations, and detailed descriptions of foods Quantification of intake imprecise due to poor recall or use of standard portion sizes	Reflects a single day's intake rather than usual intake (not a valid estimate of an individual's usual intake); several or many days over a defined time period are required to estimate usual nutrient intake Number of days needed to estimate usual intake depends on desired precision of estimate Provides quantitative estimates of foods and nutrients Tends to underestimate energy intake Provides information on food details and food preparation methods for single days of intake

Food Record	Food Frequency Questionnaire (FFQ)
The respondent (or proxy for a child) records all foods and beverages, food descriptions including preparation and ingredients, and food amounts for a specified period of time, typically recorded as consecutive 3, 7, or 14 d, but can also be nonconsecutive daily records over a period of time	The respondent (or a proxy for a child) completes a questionnaire that asks about the frequency of consumption of foods and beverages over a specified period (1 mo, 3 mo, or 1 yr); may or may not ask about portion sizes Usually self-administered
One-day records kept intermittently over a year may reflect an individual's usual intake Multiple records may be required to estimate usual nutrient intake Provides quantitative estimates of foods and nutrients Tends to underestimate energy intake Foods eaten away from home are less accurately described than those eaten at home	Useful to assess qualitative intake and dietary patterns Designed to estimate usual intake of foods; semiquantitative methods are used to estimate nutrients from food frequency information; useful for estimating foods that are consumed frequently, infrequently, or never Difficult to estimate intake of individual food items when foods are grouped Provides little information on food preparation methods or specific details about foods Tends to overestimate energy and some nutrients (extremely high nutrient estimates are not uncommon) Nutrient estimates often require adjustment for caloric intake

continued

TABLE 5-1 Continued

Criterion or Characteristic	Diet History	24-Hour Diet Recall
Validity (accuracy)	Validity is difficult to assess since intakes cannot be independently observed; recall period may be difficult for subject to conceptualize; less error from within-person variability, but error of methods has not been quantified	Standardized methodology available; provides valid estimates of mean nutrient intakes for groups, but not for individuals Well-defined time period; accuracy depends on subject's or proxy's recall or memory Does not alter person's dietary habits Portion sizes may be difficult to estimate accurately; may be more difficult to assess young children's diets since more than one proxy respondent may be required to report the day's intake completely Potential for systematic bias
Reliability (reproducibility)	Recall of past diet may be influenced by current diet Higher energy intakes in first vs. subsequent administrations in children ages 5–18 yr Repeated diet history shown to be reproducible based on 1-mo diet history and 24-h urinary nitrogen excretion	Day-to-day variability in an individual's intake reduces reliability of a single day's or few days' intake

Food Record	Food Frequency Questionnaire (FFQ)
Captures more than one day of intake	More useful for qualitative intakes rather than for quantitative intakes
Portions can be weighed or measured for improved accuracy	Calibrations with diet recalls or food records provide correlations in the range of 0.3–0.6 or 0.7 for most nutrients (mean 0.5), or 0.5–0.8 after statistical adjustment for energy and within-person variation
Validity can be improved by instruction and monitoring	
Completeness of recording decreases as the number of days increases	Eating habits are not affected by method
	Potential for systematic bias
Sequential days are not independent observations; subject may alter intake or not record all food items	
Potential for systematic bias	
Multiple days provide reliable information for less frequently consumed foods	Many types of FFQ instruments available
	Reliability is influenced by heterogeneity of population
Intraclass coefficients range from 0.5 to 0.9 for two 7-d food records	Less standardized method, especially for infants and young children
	May require subject to group foods
	Requires subject to estimate frequencies of intake
	Correlation coefficients of 0.4–0.7 for food groups and food items
	Food lists may not contain cultural foods usually eaten
	Many FFQs have been calibrated (rather than validated) against other methods; some FFQs have been tested against biomarkers
	Higher energy intakes in first vs. subsequent administrations in children ages 5–18 yr; portion sizes may be unreliable

continued

TABLE 5-1 Continued

Criterion or Characteristic	Diet History	24-Hour Diet Recall
Issues relevant to WIC populations	Requires a knowledgeable proxy respondent to describe infants' and preschoolers' diets Since infants' and young children's diets can be variable from day-to-day, it may be difficult for a proxy respondent to accurately estimate intake over a certain period of time	Difficult to estimate total intake among breast-fed infants Infants' and preschoolers' intakes may require multiple proxy respondents to completely capture all foods eaten at home, day care, preschool, and other places throughout the day Overweight adolescent and adult females tend to underreport total energy intake Standardized methodology facilitates capturing ethnic foods and food preparation methods
Respondent burden	High respondent burden Takes much more time than other methods to administer Respondents must be highly cooperative Does not require literacy if administered by trained interviewer	Low respondent burden Requires less effort on the part of the subject High response rates
Resource requirements	High Requires highly trained interviewers	Medium/high depending upon whether recall is computer-assisted and computer-coded Procedure can be administered by telephone
Administration time	1 h or more	20–30 min, on average

Food Record	Food Frequency Questionnaire (FFQ)
May be more difficult to use with low socioeconomic groups, recent immigrants, or young children May require multiple proxy respondents to record all foods eaten at home, day care, preschool, and other places throughout the day, leading to incomplete records	Food list may not contain the foods consumed by cultural or ethnic groups and be an incomplete list for the individual Commonly used FFQs have been developed more for the general population and major subgroups, and may not be appropriate for all cultural dietary patterns Extreme reporting by the individual (characterized as very high or very low energy intakes) may render the instrument useless for about 20% of individuals Overestimates energy intake by 50% in children ages 4–6 yr
High respondent burden Requires much effort and accuracy by subject Subject must be literate; poorer response rates compared with diet recall and FFQ	Low to medium respondent burden, depending on length and whether self-administered High response rates
Medium/high Procedure can be automated Requires more editing and processing time compared with diet recall	Low Does not require highly trained interviewers May be self-administered May be scored with automated procedures or optically scanned
Depends on number of days recorded and subject's abilities	10–15 min, on average for 60–75 item FFQ

TABLE 5-2 Dietary Studies Conducted in the Low-Income or WIC Population

Criterion or Characteristic	Blum et al. (1999)	Suitor et al. (1989)
WIC population	1- to 5-year-olds in North Dakota WIC program	Low-income pregnant women ages 14–43 yr in Massachusetts
Sample size and characteristics	$n = 131$ Native Americans; $n = 102$ whites; half 1–2 yr and half 3–5 yr	$n = 295$ with food frequency questionnaire (FFQ) ($n = 95$ with three diet recalls) English-speaking
Dietary method	84-item Harvard Service FFQ completed twice by parents compared to three 24-h telephone recalls over the same 4 wk using the Nutrition Data System	FFQ and subset with a second FFQ and three 24-h recalls
Major findings	Correlation coefficients ranged from 0.26 to 0.63 for nutrients (average 0.52) after adjustment for energy and within-person variability; 6% excluded due to very high or very low calories on the Harvard Service FFQ	Adjusted correlation coefficients exceeded 0.5 except for vitamin A; women who greatly overestimated intake on FFQ were at increased risk of low intake based on average of three diet recalls
Comments	Telephone recalls used with most respondents; some recalls collected in person; authors do not report on differences due to telephone or in-person administration; 86% response rate; nutrient data included supplements which may have contributed to higher correlations in this subgroup	Studies eight nutrients (energy, protein, calcium, iron, zinc, vitamins A, B_6, and C); overestimation of food occurred for about 20% of the population

Freeman, Sullivan, and Co. (1994)	Wei et al. (1999)
Children and pregnant, breastfeeding, and postpartum WIC participants	Low-income pregnant women ages 14–43 yr Massachusetts
n = 94 children and 235 women; about 1/3 each African American, Hispanic, and white	n = 101 representative sample of population from Suitor et al. citation above with diet recall
Either Block FFQ or Harvard Service FFQ (for past 4 wk) compared with three 24-h telephone recalls (for past 2–5 wk) in children ages 1–4.9 years	Pregnancy FFQ and two or three 24-h recalls over 1 mo
Correlations with diet recalls and comparison by quartile differed by racial/ethnic group; most correlations were lower than 0.5; results were generally higher for Block than for Harvard Service FFQ; neither FFQ was judged satisfactory for Hispanics or for children	Expanded eight nutrients in Suitor citation to mean intakes of 25 nutrients Unadjusted correlations ranged from 0.28 to 0.61 (mean 0.47); correlations adjusted for day-to-day variation and energy intake were 0.07 to 0.90 (mean 0.47)
African Americans and whites completed the FFQ in less than 10 min, Hispanics in less than 15 min; other mode effects of recall administration may not have been captured in this study	Excluded 14% of women with intakes above 4,500 calories Misclassification highest for saturated fat and polyunsaturated fat

use of a food frequency instrument to assess *nutrient* intake in the clinic setting. When comparing results for nutrient intakes, correlations between the FFQ and sets of diet recalls are similar to or lower than those reported by studies conducted with more advantaged populations (e.g., see Table 5-1).

Sources of Error in Dietary Methods

The validity of a diet method depends on the use of a standardized methodology, the interviewer's skill, and the subject's ability to report intake accurately. The reliability or reproducibility of a diet method relates to actual within-person variability in intake as well as to measurement error. Measurement error may be introduced by the subject, the interviewer, the methodology (such as the food measurement aids used to estimate portion size), and functions such as food coding. Bias may be caused by the systematic underreporting, overreporting, or omission of foods by an individual; interviewing or scoring processes; or errors in the food composition database used to code the dietary intake data. Discussion of some important sources of error follows.

Day-to-Day Variation

The major source of random error is day-to-day variation in intake, described earlier in this chapter (see earlier section, "A Focus on Usual Intake"). Because of high day-to-day variation in intake, high reliability (e.g., 0.8 or greater) of the diet recall or food record method would require many days of intake data. The number of days varies by the nutrient and frequency of consumption of food items containing the nutrient (Basiotis et al., 1987; IOM, 2000a; Nelson et al., 1989; Sempos et al., 1985). The error introduced by within-person variation is so large that it rules out the usefulness of a single diet recall or diet record as a method of estimating an individual's usual intake. It appears impossible to eliminate within-person variation as a source of random error in the estimation of an individual's usual intake. Even if usual nutrient intake could be assessed with several days of observations of an individual's intake, collection of multiple days of intake is not feasible in the WIC clinic setting (see criterion 6, "Operational Constraints," in Chapter 4).

There are two approaches to minimizing within-person variability in dietary data. The first involves collecting many days of dietary intake data and averaging the data to capture usual (mean) intake as well as the precision of the estimate (standard deviation around the mean). The number of days needed to attain a usually desired level of reliability of 0.8 or higher varies by the nutrient or food group to be measured because it is directly related to the magnitude of the within-person variability (IOM, 2000a; Nelson et al., 1989). Although the errors of individuals in a group tend to cancel each other out and leave an unbiased estimate of the true value for the group, estimates of usual intake with sufficient accuracy and reliability to judge an individual's eligibility status require multiple measures of daily intake.

The second approach to minimizing within-person variability is to use an FFQ. With this method, the individual is expected to summarize the usual intake of food items, based on her knowledge of how her dietary choices vary from day to day. In this case, reliability is typically judged by assessing the reproducibility of the intake estimates from repeated administrations of the questionnaire, and validity is assessed by comparing the intake estimates with usual nutrient intakes estimated from multiple days of intake using either diet recalls or diet records.

Reliability or reproducibility of both nutrient intake and food intake may be a problem in FFQs, just as it is in diet recalls. Using FFQs, correlation coefficients of 0.4–0.7 are typical for the reliability (reproducibility) of nutrients (McPherson et al., 2000; Serdula et al., 2001; Thompson and Byers, 1994), food groups, and single food items (Ajani et al., 1994; Bohlscheid-Thomas et al., 1997; Colditz et al., 1987; Feskanich et al., 1993; Jain and McLaughlin, 2000; Jarvinen et al., 1993; Salvini et al., 1989).

In a review of the literature on diet methods for children, McPherson et al. (2000) reported on two reliability test-retests of an FFQ among adolescents. An FFQ was administered 1 year apart to 9- to 18-year-olds by Rockett and colleagues (1995). They found average correlations of 0.5 for fruits, vegetables, and fruits and vegetables combined, and higher reproducibility for girls than for boys. Frank et al. (1992) compared a 64-item FFQ administered 2 weeks apart to 12- to 17-year-olds. Two-thirds of the adolescents reported similar results for low-fat milk, diet carbonated soft drinks, and shellfish. For 12 food groups, there was 50 percent or better agreement between the two FFQs.

Underreporting and Overreporting Intake

Diet Recalls and Food Records. Table 5-1 indicates that, in affluent societies such as the United States, diet recalls and food records for adults are both subject to systematic error or bias, primarily the underreporting of energy intake (Bingham, 1987, 1991). In U.S. dietary intake surveys that use diet recalls, up to 31 percent of the subjects may underreport their intake (Briefel et al., 1995, 1997; Klesges et al., 1995a). Compared with individuals of healthy weight, overweight adults and adolescents (and those trying to lose weight) are more likely to underreport energy intakes (Briefel et al., 1997; Klesges et al., 1995a). Similarly, those with lower socioeconomic status, education, and literacy levels are more likely to underreport intake than are other groups (Briefel et al., 1995, 1997; Klesges et al., 1995a). Baranowski et al. (1991) found that mothers were more likely to underreport than to overreport their young children's food intake during 24-hour diet recalls; mothers underreported food intake 18 percent of the time and overreported food intake 10 percent of the time. Several research groups (Johnson et al., 1998; Kroke et al., 1999; Sawaya et al., 1996; Tran et al.,

2000) confirm that 24-hour diet recalls underreport energy intake when intakes are compared with estimates of energy expenditure as measured by doubly labeled water. A review of dietary assessment among preschool children found that diet recalls both overestimated and underestimated energy intake (Serdula et al., 2001). A review of dietary method studies among children ages 5–18 years also found that food records underestimated energy intake compared to doubly labeled water (McPherson et al., 2000). At present, there is no definitive way to identify individuals who either underreport or overreport their intake on diet recalls or food records—except, perhaps, in the extreme. Such systematic errors may mean that sets of diet recalls or records are questionable standards for evaluating the performance of FFQs and diet histories, but such evaluation is common practice (see below).

Food Frequency Questionnaires and Diet Histories. Previous studies of doubly labeled water in children have shown that FFQs overestimate total energy intake by about 50 percent in children (Goran, 1998; McPherson et al., 2000; Serdula et al., 2001). Kaskoun and colleagues (1994) reported that FFQs completed by parents for 4- to 6-year-old children substantially overestimate the children's energy intake by 58 percent in comparison with total energy expenditure as measured by doubly labeled water. Dietary studies using FFQs overestimated energy intake among children ages 5–18 years (McPherson et al., 2000). Taylor and Goulding (1998) found that a 35-item FFQ overestimated calcium intake by 18 percent compared with 4-day diet records based on parents' reports of the intakes of their 3- to 6-year-old children. The overestimation of intake based on long lists of foods in an FFQ is one reason that researchers statistically adjust for a group's total caloric intake when analyzing nutrient intakes from a FFQ. The usefulness of such adjustments when using a tool to establish eligibility is questionable. In addition, care must be taken to not overadjust (Thompson and Byers, 1994). Dietary histories also were found to overestimate energy intake by 12 percent in a small group of 3-year-old children and by 8 percent of 5-year-old children compared to the doubly labeled water method (Serdula et al., 2001). Therefore, using a diet history method to assess an individual's dietary risk for WIC eligibility would be biased toward higher estimates of energy, food, and nutrients. Using a diet assessment tool that overestimates intake would result in falsely classifying many individuals as meeting the *Dietary Guidelines* or having intakes that exceed a cut-off point for nutrient intake.

Differences by Type of Food. Several investigators (e.g., Feskanich et al., 1993; Salvini et al., 1989; Worsley et al., 1984) reported that people tend to overestimate their intake of foods perceived as healthy (such as vegetables) and underreport foods considered to be less healthy. Bingham (1987) suggested that fat, sugar, and alcohol are most subject to underreporting; however, there are no definitive conclusions about systematic errors related to specific foods or dietary patterns (Schoeller, 1990; Tarasuk, 1996; Tarasuk and Brooker, 1997). A tendency to overreport vegetables and underreport sources of fat, sugar, and alcohol would lead to overestimation of intake of one food group and some essential nutrients and to underestimation of energy. These inaccuracies could result in a low specificity. That is, people who truly do not meet criteria based on the *Dietary Guidelines* or nutrient cut-off points would be misclassified as ineligible for WIC.

Portion Size Estimation

Diet recalls and food records are subject to respondents' errors in reporting or recalling portion sizes consumed. Weighed food records provide more accurate portion size data, but weighing requires additional time and effort by the subject. In a series of experiments investigating the cognitive processes involved in long-term recall, Smith (1991) studied the ability of subjects to recall or distinguish portion sizes accurately. He found that individuals cannot distinguish between the definitions of portion size provided by commonly used FFQs (for example, small, medium, or large; or medium = 1 medium apple). This research suggests that individuals have poor ability to provide accurate portion size information and that typical food frequency instruments are not satisfactory for collecting high-quality information on portion sizes. This limits the usefulness of FFQs in quantifying the numbers of standard servings of food consumed or nutrient intakes by individuals—thus increasing the chance of misclassifying a person's WIC eligibility status.

Interviewer Bias

The person collecting the dietary intake data may introduce systematic error by assuming certain cultural practices rather than asking the subject, or by using unstandardized, leading probes to elicit information. In the research setting, controls ordinarily are in place to minimize these problems. In a service setting, however, there may be interruptions, distractions, time constraints, and minimally trained staff collecting dietary intake information.

The Accuracy of Food Frequency Questionnaires

Correlations with Usual Intake from Diet Recalls or Food Records—Adolescents and Adults

FFQs have many features that make them seem attractive for dietary data collection in WIC settings (Table 5-1), but do they reduce within-person variation and other sources of error enough that a valid result can be obtained in a short time? To examine the validity of FFQs, investigators often compare results from an FFQ with the estimation of usual intake obtained from a set of research-quality diet recalls or food records. They estimate usual intake of the individuals in the group by obtaining 24-hour recalls or food records over many days using standardized methods. The results are sometimes called a gold standard against which the accuracy of other methods can be compared, despite the possibility of systematic underreporting as mentioned above.

Correlations between estimates from FFQs and two 7-day records are typically in the range of 0.3 to 0.6 for most nutrients (Sempos et al., 1992). After statistical adjustments (deattenuation) for energy intake and within-person variation using data from diet recalls or diet records, correlations reported for FFQs used in research studies range between 0.4 and 0.8 (Block et al., 1990; Blum et al., 1999; Brown et al., 1996; Friis et al., 1997; Robinson et al., 1996; Stein et al., 1992; Suitor et al., 1989; Treiber et al., 1990; Willett et al., 1987). Mean correlation coefficients cluster around 0.5 (Jain and McLaughlin, 2000; Jain et al., 1996; Longenecker et al., 1993). In general, correlations for adolescents between the validation standard and diet method were higher for single diet recalls and diet records than for FFQs (McPherson et al., 2000). In one study among adolescents, correlations between 3-day diet records and serum micronutrients ranged from 0.32 to 0.65 (McPherson et al., 2000).

The nutrients being assessed and the number of items on an FFQ can affect the validity of the questionnaire. A 15-item questionnaire designed to determine the adequacy only of calcium intake had a 0.8 correlation with intake determined from a 4-day food record (Angus et al., 1989). Among tools that assessed a broad range of nutrients, the highest correlation coefficients that the committee found for women were those reported by the EPIC Group of Spain (1997) for a 50- to 60-minute diet history interview compared with 24-hour recalls obtained over the previous year. Excluding cholesterol, the correlations ranged from 0.51 for β-carotene to 0.83 for alcohol; half were 0.7 or greater. However, even a correlation coefficient of 0.8 reflects a substantial degree of error when examined at the level of the individual (see "Agreement of Results by Quartile and Misclassification," below).

Wei et al. (1999) reported on the use of a modified FFQ to assess nutrients in low-income pregnant women ages 14 to 43 years (see Table 5-2). Fourteen percent of the sample was excluded due to unusually high intakes (above 4,500 calories) indicating probable overestimation problems for a proportion of the population. Unadjusted correlation coefficients ranged from 0.3 for carotene to 0.6 for folate, with a mean correlation coefficient of 0.47, following exclusions.

The validity of questionnaires with regard to food or food group intake also is a problem. Little evidence is available concerning the ability of FFQs to estimate intake correctly when servings of foods or food groups (rather than nutrients) are the units of comparison (Thompson et al., 2000). In the study by Bohlscheid-Thomas and colleagues (1997), correlation coefficients between food group intakes obtained from the 24-hour recalls and a subsequent FFQ ranged from 0.14 for legumes to 0.9 for alcoholic beverages. For 9 food groups, correlations were less than 0.4, for 11 they were between 0.4 and 0.6, and for 4 they were greater than 0.6. Similarly, Feskanich and coworkers (1993) reported a range of 0.17 for "other nuts" to 0.95 for "bananas," with a mean correlation of 0.6 after adjusting for within-person variation in intake. Field et al. (1998) found correlations of 0.1 to 0.3 for vegetables, fruit juices, and fruits, and 0.4 for fruits and vegetables combined among ninth to twelfth graders between a 27-item FFQ and an average of three diet recalls. In general, these correlation coefficients are not better than those found by investigators studying nutrients rather than foods.

Correlations with Usual Intake from Diet Recalls or Food Records—Young Children

Few validity studies have been conducted of questionnaires designed to assess the diets of young children (Baranowski et al., 1991; Blum et al., 1999; Goran et al., 1998; McPherson et al., 2000; Persson and Carlgren, 1984). Blum et al. (1999) assessed the validity of the Harvard Service FFQ in Native American and Caucasian children 1 to 5 years of age in the North Dakota WIC Program (see Table 5-2). An 84-item FFQ was self-administered twice by parents, at the first WIC visit and then after the completion of three 24-hour recalls. Correlations ranged from 0.26 for fiber to 0.63 for magnesium and averaged 0.5.

Persson and Carlgren (1984) evaluated various dietary assessment techniques in a study of Swedish infants and children. They found that a short FFQ (asked of parents) was a poor screening instrument with systematic biases when used for 4-year-olds. Staple foods such as potatoes, bread, cheese, and fruits were overestimated and sucrose-rich foods such as cakes were underestimated compared with results from food records.

Agreement of Results by Quantile and Misclassification

A number of researchers question the appropriateness of using the correlation coefficient (Hebert and Miller, 1991; Liu, 1994) or a single type of correlation coefficient (Negri et al., 1994) to assess the validity and reliability of food-based questionnaires because a high correlation does not necessarily mean high agreement. This question is especially relevant to the situation in WIC, where estimation errors are of great concern if they result in the misclassification of individuals with regard to their dietary risk. Another way to examine validity and the potential misclassification problem is to examine results of studies that report agreement of the results by quantile.

Robinson et al. (1996) compared results from a 4-day diet record obtained at 16 weeks of gestation with those from a 100-item FFQ obtained at 15 weeks of gestation. They found a range: 30 percent of the women were classified in the same quartile of intake for starch, and 41 percent were in the same quartile for

TABLE 5-3 Probabilities of Misclassification of a Reference Ranking in Quintiles, Using an Imperfect Alternative

Absolute Difference in Quintile Rank	P				
	0.95	0.9	0.8	0.7	0.6
0	0.674	0.573	0.467	0.403	0.357
1	0.315	0.378	0.403	0.400	0.390
2	0.011	0.047	0.113	0.156	0.184
3	0.000	0.002	0.016	0.037	0.060
4	0.000	0.000	0.001	0.003	0.009

SOURCE: Walker and Blettner (1985).

calcium. Eight percent were classified in opposite quartiles for energy, protein, and vitamin E intakes. Friis et al. (1997) found that 71 percent of young women were in the same quintile or within one quintile when comparing intakes from an FFQ and three sets of 4-day food records. On average, 3.8 percent were grossly misclassified into the highest and lowest quintiles by the two methods.

Freeman, Sullivan, et al. (1994) compared a 4-week FFQ (either the Block FFQ or the Harvard Service FFQ) with three 24-hour diet recalls conducted by telephone among 94 children and 235 women participating in WIC (see Table 5-2). Most correlations between the FFQ and the average of three recalls were below 0.5. The FFQ performed more poorly among children than among women and also among Hispanics than among African Americans and non-Hispanic whites.

Suitor et al. (1989) compared the results of three 24-hour dietary recalls and a 90-item FFQ among pregnant women and found that fewer than half of the women who were in the lowest quintile by one method also were in the lowest quintile by the other method (see Table 5-2). The quintile agreement ranged from 27 percent for iron to 54 percent for calcium. Percentage agreement improved (to 43 percent for protein and to 77 percent for calcium) when individuals from the first and second quintile of the FFQ were compared with those in the first quintile of the 24-hour dietary recalls. Clearly, substantial misclassification of nutrient intake occurred at the individual level.

Different questionnaires give different results with the same subjects (McCann et al., 1999; Wirfalt et al., 1998). Although McCann and colleagues (1999) reported that the results of different methods are correlated (i.e., r ranges from 0.29 to 0.80), the methods would likely classify individuals differently. Walker and Blettner (1985) examined potential agreement when results from an imperfect method of dietary assessment (e.g., an FFQ) are compared with those from a method believed to be accurate (e.g., many days of research-quality food records). Table 5-3 shows their calculations of the probabilities of misclassification in quintile ranking for correlation coefficients ranging from 0.0 to 0.95.

0.5	0.4	0.3	0.2	0.1	0.0
0.321	0.290	0.263	0.240	0.219	0.200
0.379	0.367	0.355	0.344	0.332	0.320
0.203	0.216	0.225	0.232	0.234	0.240
0.081	0.101	0.118	0.134	0.148	0.160
0.017	0.027	0.038	0.051	0.065	0.080

Note that even if the correlation coefficient between the two methods were 0.8 (ordinarily considered to be excellent correspondence), less than half of all respondents would be allocated to the same quintile by the two methods. This indicates that FFQs hold great potential for misclassification at the level of the individual—regardless of whether nutrient, food, or food group intakes are being estimated.

Another way to examine the error in misclassification would be to consider the sensitivity and specificity of the tool and how they would translate to numbers of people miscategorized. Using the relatively high sensitivity and specificity values from the example in the following section and assuming that 25 percent of the population meets the *Dietary Guidelines* (a value much higher than currently estimated), we see in Table 5-4 that roughly one-fourth of the population (275/1,000 individuals) would be misclassified. Increasing the sensitivity by increasing the cut-off would increase the number of eligible individuals who test positive and reduce misclassification. If a lower, more realistic value representing the percentage of the population that meets the *Dietary Guidelines* were used, the percent of eligible persons who would be found ineligible would be larger (Table 5-5).

Limitations and Uses of Brief Dietary Methods

Shortening and simplifying FFQs may make it easier for WIC clientele to respond (whether the FFQ is self-administered or administered by WIC personnel) (Subar et al., 1995), but is the validity of short FFQs acceptable? Based on studies by Byers et al. (1985), Caan et al. (1995), Haile et al. (1986), and others, it is unreasonable to expect that a shortened FFQ will be more accurate than a longer version. For example, Caan et al. (1995) evaluated the sensitivity, specificity, and positive predictive value of a 15-item fat screener when used to identify persons with total fat intakes greater than 38 percent of calories. When they compared results with those obtained from the 60-item Health Habits and

TABLE 5-4 Results from a Dietary Tool with a Relatively High Sensitivity and Specificity when 25 percent of the Population Meets the *Dietary Guidelines*

	Result from Dietary Tool		
	Eligible	Ineligible	Total
Does not meet the *Dietary Guidelines*	563	187	750
Meets the *Dietary Guidelines*	88	162	250
Total	651	349	1,000

NOTE: Assumptions: sensitivity = 75%, specificity = 65%.

TABLE 5-5 Results from a Dietary Tool with a Relatively High Sensitivity and Specificity when 5 percent of the Population Meets the *Dietary Guidelines*

	Result from Dietary Tool		
	Eligible	Ineligible	Total
Does not meet the *Dietary Guidelines*	713	237	950
Meets the *Dietary Guidelines*	17	33	50
Total	730	270	1,000

NOTE: Assumptions: sensitivity = 75%, specificity = 65%.

History Questionnaire (Block et al., 1990), the fat screener had a low rate (2.7 percent) of gross misclassification—for example, the rate when the lowest quintile by the FFQ was compared with the highest two quintiles by the screener. Caan and colleagues (1995) found that the fat screener had insufficient sensitivity and specificity to be used as a single assessment method for fat. For example, when sensitivity was 75 percent, specificity was 65 percent; but when the cut-off point was raised, sensitivity was 47 percent and specificity was 89 percent. They suggested that the screener would be useful in combination with other dietary methods that also estimate energy intake.

Others have found that measures taken to shorten and simplify questionnaires reduce their validity in the research setting. For example, Schaffer and colleagues (1997) reported that median energy intake from a shortened telephone version of an FFQ was 23 percent lower in women than that obtained from a longer FFQ. These investigators reported correlation coefficients ranging from 0.45 for vitamin E to 0.78 for fiber for the two FFQs, suggesting considerable lack of agreement. Similarly, Thompson and coworkers (2000) reported that both a 7-item and a 16-item screener for fruit and vegetable consumption underestimate intake.

Brief dietary tools have varying degrees of usefulness, depending upon the need for quantitative, qualitative, or behavioral data. They have been developed to measure usual intake, to screen for high intakes of certain nutrients (e.g., total fat, iron, calcium), or to measure usual intake of particular food groups (such as fruits and vegetables). Several examples have been published (e.g., Block et al., 1989; Caan et al., 1995; Feskanich et al., 1993; Kristal et al., 1990; McPherson et al., 2000; NCHS, 1994; Thompson and Byers, 1994). A major limitation of using them to assess intake in the WIC clinic is that they usually target one nutrient or food group, rather than the entire diet. Thus, they are not directly relevant to determining whether the individual met the *Dietary Guidelines* or consumed an adequate diet, but they may be useful for planning targeted nutrition education.

METHODS TO COMPARE FOOD INTAKES WITH THE *DIETARY GUIDELINES*

The committee was given the charge of investigating methods to determine if an individual fails to meet the *Dietary Guidelines*. For example, can a practical, accurate method be found or developed to compare reported food intake with recommendations derived from the *Dietary Guidelines* (USDA/HHS, 2000). The committee found no studies that directly examine the performance of dietary intake tools used to compare an individual's food intake with the *Dietary Guidelines*, but did find the following related information.

Dietary Intake Form Method

Strohmeyer and colleagues (1984) claimed that a rapid dietary screening device (called the Dietary Intake Form, or DIF) " . . . provides a rapid, valid, reliable, and acceptable method of identifying the individual with a poor diet" (p. 428). Although the DIF was developed before the existence of the *Dietary Guidelines* and the Food Guide Pyramid, it was intended to compare a person's intake with reference values that are similar to the Pyramid's five food group recommendations. The DIF asks the person to write the number of times the following foods are consumed per week: yogurt and milk; cheese; fish, eggs, meat; dried peas and beans; leafy green vegetables; citrus fruit; other fruits and vegetables; bread; and noodles, grains, and cereals. It also asks the respondent to circle his or her portion size as it compares with specified standards. The average time to complete the DIF is about 4.5 minutes, with a range of 2 to 10 minutes.[5] A staff member computes a DIF score by a series of arithmetic processes.

The methods that Strohmeyer and colleagues used to test reliability and validity are of questionable relevance to the WIC setting. They tested reliability

---

[5] It is notable that 21 percent of the subjects did not complete the forms; reasons were not reported.

using 40 college students who completed the DIF on two occasions 2 weeks apart. Correlation coefficients for the paired food-group and total dietary scores averaged 0.81. Validity testing involved input by researchers rather than by clients and scoring by researchers rather than by clinic staff. Researchers entered data from 29 8-day food diaries onto DIFs and then computed dietary scores. Subsequently, they correlated those DIF scores with total mean Nutrient Adequacy Ratios (NAR, in which NAR equals the subject's daily intake of a nutrient divided by the Recommended Dietary Allowance of that nutrient). Under these carefully controlled conditions, the correlation of DIF and NAR scores was 0.83. It is likely that reliability and validity testing using the clinic population and clinic personnel would produce less favorable results. More importantly, the limitations described for brief FFQs would be applicable to the DIF as well.

Mean Adequacy Ratio Methods

A more recent study examined the sensitivity and specificity of two Pyramid-based methods of scoring nutritional adequacy (Schuette et al., 1996). For both scoring methods, registered dietitians obtained data from 1-day food records. They assigned the reported food items to the five Pyramid food groups and "other" (fats, oils, sugars). In the first method, the score represents the number of food groups from which the person consumed at least the minimum recommended number of servings. In the second method, the score represents the number of food groups from which the person consumed at least one serving. The two types of scores were compared with a mean adequacy ratio (MAR-5)[6] based on the subject's intakes of iron, calcium, magnesium, vitamin A, and vitamin B_6 as calculated from the same food record. For the first method, sensitivity was 99 percent but specificity was only 16 percent. That is, the first food group method classified nutritionally inadequate diets as inadequate, but it had extremely low ability to classify nutritionally adequate diets as adequate. For the second method, sensitivity was 89 percent and specificity was 45 percent. Thus, even when the cut-off point was more lenient (as in the second method) the ability to identify the nutritionally adequate diets was no better than chance. Either MAR method would depend on data from one or two 24-hour diet recalls, and thus would be subject to all the limitations of diet recalls presented earlier in this chapter.

---

[6] MAR-5 = average nutrient adequacy ratio (NAR) of the five nutrients. NAR is the nutrient content calculated as a percentage of the RDA and truncated at 100.

Estimating the Number of Pyramid Portions

Accuracy of Estimation

The portion sizes that an individual consumes can make a great difference in the degree to which his or her intake meets the recommendations made in the Food Guide Pyramid. Questionnaires either assume a standard portion size, which may or may not be shown on the questionnaire,[7] or the respondent is asked to choose a single average portion size (small, medium, or large). However, two major factors affect the accuracy of portion size estimation: (1) within-person variability in portion size, and (2) ability to recall portion size (see earlier section, "Portion Size Estimation").

Within-person variability in portion size is greater than between-person variability for most foods and for all the food groups studied by Hunter et al. (1988). That is, for food groups, the range of the variance ratios (within/between) obtained from four 1-week diet records was 1.6 (fruit) to 4.8 (meat) when pizza was excluded (the variance ratio was 22 for pizza). No studies were found that examine the extent to which the portion size used on a questionnaire reflects the individual's average portion size.

Using the U.S. Department of Agriculture Protocol for Portion Sizes

Even if portion size has been reported accurately, the consumption of mixed foods complicates the estimation of the number of portions a person consumes from each of the five Pyramid food groups. For example, 1 cup of some kinds of breakfast cereal may be about half grain and half sugar by weight so should be counted as only one-half serving from the breads and cereals food group.

To determine the numbers of servings of foods in the five major food groups from diet recalls or records accurately, researchers at the U.S. Department of Agriculture (USDA) developed the Continuing Survey of Food Intake by Individuals (CSFII) Pyramid Servings database (Cleveland et al., 1997). Eighty-nine percent of the foods in this database are multiple-ingredient foods. USDA separated these foods into their ingredients and categorized these ingredients into food groups that were consistent with Pyramid definitions for serving sizes (USDA, 1992). If a woman reported eating chicken pie, for example, the database allows estimation of the servings or fractions of a serving of grains, meat, vegetables, and milk products (if applicable) provided by the specified weight of the pie. This means that the accurate comparison of food group intake with recommended intake would require accurate food intake data collected over a number of independent days together with computerized assignment of food ingredients to food groups. Notably, this method of estimating servings was

---

[7] Often the portion size used is either the median for the population group as obtained from a nationwide survey or a common unit such as one slice of bread.

used in two rigorous studies that found that fewer than 1 percent of women (Krebs-Smith et al., 1997) and young children (Munoz et al., 1997) met recommendations for all five food groups (see Chapter 8).

Healthy Eating Index Scores

USDA's Center for Nutrition Policy and Promotion developed the Healthy Eating Index (HEI) to assess and monitor the dietary status of Americans (Kennedy et al., 1995). The 10 components of the HEI represent different aspects of a healthful diet. Five of the components cover the five food groups from the Food Guide Pyramid and the other five cover elements of the 1995 *Dietary Guidelines* concerning fat, saturated fat, cholesterol, sodium, and variety. The computation of the number of servings from each food group requires the use of complex computerized methods to disaggregate mixed foods into ingredients (Cleveland et al., 1997). Each component may receive a maximum score of 10. The index yields a single score (the maximum score is 100) covering diet as a whole and measuring "how well the diets of all Americans conform to the recommendations of the Dietary Guidelines and the Food Guide Pyramid" (Variyam et al., 1998).

Theoretically, an HEI score would be a comprehensive indicator of whether a potential WIC participant of at least 2 years of age *fails to meet Dietary Guidelines*. However, the complexity of methods required to obtain this score limits the feasibility of using it in the WIC setting. The process described above must be used to separate foods into ingredients and categorize the ingredients into food groups, and separate scores must be computed for each of the 10 components of the HEI score.

An HEI score of 100 is equivalent to meeting all the Food Guide Pyramid recommendations plus recommendations for fat, saturated fat, cholesterol, and sodium.[8] According to Bowman and colleagues (1998), a score of more than 80 implies a "good" diet. Using 1994–1996 CSFII data, approximately 12 percent of the population had a good diet. A good ranking, based on an HEI score of 80, is considerably more lenient than a criterion in which intake of fewer than the recommended number of servings in the Food Guide Pyramid is the cut-off for *failure to meet Dietary Guidelines*. Even if an HEI score could be obtained accurately in the WIC setting, the score would likely be sensitive, but not specific. The HEI score could be no more accurate than the data from which it is derived. Thus, it is subject to the limitations of the diet recall or FFQ used.

---

[8] The HEI also includes a variety score, but it is not applicable to the current *Dietary Guidelines*.

CONCLUSIONS REGARDING FOOD-BASED DIETARY ASSESSMENT METHODS FOR ELIGIBILITY DETERMINATION

Under the best circumstances in a research setting, dietary assessment tools are not accurate for individuals. In particular, a diet recall or food record cannot provide a sufficiently accurate estimate of usual food or nutrient intake to avoid extensive misclassification. Similarly, research-quality FFQs result in substantial misclassification of individuals in a group when results from FFQs are compared with those from sets of diet recalls or food records. Moreover, studies by Bowman et al. (1998), Krebs-Smith et al. (1997), McCullough et al. (2000), and Munoz et al. (1997) (see Chapter 8) suggested that even if the use of research methods were possible in the WIC setting, such methods would identify nearly everyone as *failing to meet Dietary Guidelines*.

In WIC, a dietary assessment method is used by the competent professional authority (CPA) to determine an individual's eligibility for WIC in the event that the person has no anthropometric, medical, or biochemical risks (see Chapter 2). The result thus may determine whether or not the applicant will receive WIC benefits for a period of several months or longer. Ordinarily, the CPA compares the individual's reported intake of foods with preset standards for the numbers of servings in five or more food groups. Even if reported intakes were accurate, estimation of food group scores would likely be inaccurate because of the high frequency of mixed foods. If reported intake or assigned food group scores are inaccurate, correct identification of eligibility status is compromised.

Shortening FFQs tends to decrease their validity. Very short screens are targeted to one nutrient or food group rather than providing a relatively complete assessment of dietary intake. Methods to compare food intakes with dietary guidance have the limitations of short screens or are too complex to be useful in the WIC setting. Environmental and other factors present in the WIC setting are expected to decrease the validity of tools when compared with those found in the research setting. Consequently, the validity reported for research-quality FFQs can be considered an upper limit for the validity of questionnaires used by WIC.

When using these dietary assessment procedures for group assessment, researchers generally have been willing to tolerate a substantial amount of error, for which they could partially compensate by increasing the number of participants in their research or using statistical correction procedures, called corrections for attenuation (Traub, 1994). Error in the assessment of an individual for certification in the WIC program (that is, misclassification error), however, has serious consequences: truly eligible individuals may not be classified as eligible for the services (less than perfect *sensitivity*), or individuals not truly eligible for the services may receive them (less than perfect *specificity*).

Because of these limitations, the committee concludes that there are not now, nor will there likely ever be, dietary assessment methods that are both sufficiently valid and practical to distinguish individuals who are ineligible from those eligible for WIC based on the criterion *failure to meet Dietary Guidelines* or based on cut-off points for nutrient intake. Nonetheless, dietary tools have an important role in WIC in planning or targeting nutrition education for WIC clients, as described in Chapter 9.

6

Assessment of Physical Activity

As with dietary assessment (see Chapter 5), there are many challenges in the valid and reliable assessment of physical activity in individuals. This is especially true in the populations served by WIC to whom the *Dietary Guidelines* would apply—children ages 2 to 5 years and pregnant or postpartum women. This chapter describes the challenges and summarizes what is currently known about the patterns of physical activity in these populations and the methods available for assessing their physical activity. It makes recommendations about the role of physical activity assessment in the WIC program and about future research needs in this area.

CHALLENGES IN ASSESSING PHYSICAL ACTIVITY

Physical Activity in Preschoolers

The *Dietary Guidelines* and thus the physical activity guideline contained within them, apply only to children 2 years of age and older. There are no published guidelines for activity in children 12 to 23 months of age. While the *Dietary Guidelines* recommend 60 minutes of "moderate" daily physical activity for 2- to 5-year-old children, there is not a definition provided of what constitutes moderate activity for children.

Direct observation of activity is the best criterion measure for any instrument to assess physical activity in children 2 to 5 years of age. Such observations reveal that as children play, they have short and intermittent, rather than continuous, bouts of activity with frequent rest periods (Bailey et al., 1995).

These bouts rarely last more than 10 minutes. This difference in activity patterns between adults and children is also seen in many animal species. The difference is thought to result from differing needs of the developing brain to provide itself, through activity, with a pattern of stimulation from the environment that subserves its own optimal development (Rowland, 1998). Compared to adults, children have more spontaneous activity, a shorter attention span, less interest in sustaining a single activity, more interest in trying new activities, and the need for more frequent rest periods. Therefore, assessing physical activity in young children, as compared to adults, requires child-specific definitions of what constitutes moderate physical activity. Furthermore, children 2 to 5 years of age are not cognitively capable of recalling their own physical activity in terms of activity type, frequency, duration, or intensity. This is analogous to the inability of children this age to recall sufficient details of their own dietary intake for a valid assessment of diet. Thus, as with dietary assessment, parent (or other adult caretaker) reporting is required, which poses other challenges to conducting valid assessment of physical activity.

Physical Activity in Women

Much of the physical activity of women of child-bearing age, especially those already raising young children, occurs in the context of walking for transportation, the workplace, childcare, and household tasks, rather than in leisure-time physical activity (Ainsworth, 2000a, 2000b; Eyler et al., 1998; Masse et al., 1998). Thus, many self-report measures developed for adults (and many with a focus on men) do not contain the necessary questions about nonleisure-time physical activity that would allow for a full accounting of the activity of many women. This appears especially true for ethnic minorities and women with young children, such as those receiving WIC services, who are reported in many physical activity surveys to have very low levels of leisure-time physical activity and who appear quite sedentary. These women, however, may be involved in moderate physical activity while doing things such as household chores, walking at work, taking care of children or other family members, shopping, and gardening (Ainsworth et al., 1999).

Any physical activity assessment tool aimed at accurately classifying physical activity levels in women enrolled in the WIC program would need to include a variety of activities performed by these women in their everyday lives. For example, including household activities in physical activity questionnaires has been shown to dramatically alter the classification of women's activity levels in relationship to men (Ainsworth et al., 1993b). However, capturing women's moderate-intensity physical activity with several brief questions may be an insurmountable challenge for some of the same reasons that it is with preschool children. For women and young children, many of these moderate-intensity activities occur outside of structured settings, in short bouts, and admixed with other activities of lesser intensity (Masse et al., 1998). Activities are quite varied and differ among women by age and ethnicity (e.g., the lesser role of walking in urban African-American women than in rural Native-American women [Ainsworth et al., 1999]). Thus, it is not clear which or how many examples or cues should be given to prompt the recall of moderate-intensity physical activity on the brief survey questions that are aimed at making global physical activity assessments (Ainsworth, 2000a).

With regard to women who are either pregnant, postpartum, or lactating, the *Dietary Guidelines* do not make specific exclusions or modifications of the quantitative physical activity recommendation. There have been no recommendations from the American College of Obstetricians and Gynecologists (ACOG) since 1994 regarding physical activity in pregnant and postpartum women (ACOG, 1994). The 1994 ACOG recommendations stated that in uncomplicated pregnancies "there are no data in humans to indicate that pregnant women should limit exercise intensity and lower target heart rates because of potential adverse effects." While these recommendations are not quantitative, they still allow the target of "30 minutes of moderate physical activity most days of the week, preferably daily." A recent review of studies examining the maternal and fetal effects of maternal exercise during pregnancy suggests that even strenuous exercise regimens are associated with improved outcomes for mother and fetus (Clapp, 2000). In summary, there is no evidence or conflicting "expert" recommendation suggesting that the quantitative physical activity guideline in the *Dietary Guidelines* does not apply to pregnant, postpartum, or lactating women who are not experiencing medical complications of these physiologic states.

Epidemiology of Physical Activity in the WIC Population

Published studies describing the physical activity patterns of WIC recipients are very limited. Because of the inherent difficulties with measuring physical activity in preschool children, as discussed previously, there are no available data comparing physical activity levels across socioeconomic gradients in preschool children. Even among school-age children, there is no clear evidence that children of lower socioeconomic status have lower levels of physical activity. In a recent analysis of Third National Health and Nutrition Examination Survey data, ethnic minority children (non-Hispanic blacks and Mexican Americans) who were 8 to 16 years of age reported being less physically active than non-Hispanic white children (Andersen et al., 1998). However, these activity data were not examined by family income or parental education.

In a nationally representative sample of pregnant women, the prevalence of exercise during pregnancy did not differ significantly by household income, although women with more than high school education were slightly more active (Zhang and Savitz, 1996). In a study of Pittsburgh, Pennsylvania residents that examined job-related, household, and leisure-time physical activity, Ford and colleagues (1991) noted less physical activity for women of lower socioeconomic status. This is consistent with others studies showing that activity levels are lower in adults with lower socioeconomic status (Macera and Pratt, 2000; Troiano et al., 2001), particularly as measured by educational level (Bild et al., 1993; White et al., 1987). However, these studies all focused largely on leisure-time physical activity. Only one study was identified that specifically examined physical activity levels among women enrolled in WIC, but this assessment was only for leisure-time physical activity (Jeffery and French, 1998). In that study, baseline data were reported from a weight gain prevention trial that involved both high- and low-income groups of women. The low-income women were recruited from WIC and, compared to the high-income group, tended to watch more television but did not report significantly less physical activity. In this low-income group, television viewing was strongly related to body mass index but not to physical activity.

METHODS TO ASSESS PHYSICAL ACTIVITY

Overview of Methods

Several comprehensive reviews have been written on the different methods to assess physical activity in adults and children (Baranowski et al., 1992; Goran, 1998; Kohl et al., 2000; Kriska and Caspersen, 1997; Pate, 1993; Sallis and Saelens, 2000; Welk and Wood, 2000). Of the many methods, only recall questionnaires (interviewer- or self-administered) have potential feasibility for application in WIC. All such self-report measures, including proxy reporting from parents or adult caregivers, are subject to bias. All other nonrecall methods are not feasible, primarily because of expense or burden on WIC staff or clients.

Although the committee reviewed the current dietary assessment tools used in WIC (see Chapter 2), WIC agencies were not requested to submit all general questionnaires used in WIC clinics. These general questionnaires may have also contained items on physical activity. Nonetheless, among the 54 agencies supplying assessment tools for review (dietary and/or general), none had any physical activity questions for children and only 4 had any physical activity questions for women (self-report). Only 1 state had a question about television viewing and this was aimed at children.

Assessment of physical activity involves many of the same challenges as assessment of food intake (Baranowski, 1985, 1988; Baranowski and Simons-Morton, 1991). Therefore, the committee believed it was appropriate to use the same eight criteria in the framework for evaluating tools to assess dietary risk (see Chapter 4) to evaluate each of the methods deemed potentially feasible for physical activity assessment in WIC. Thus, any suitable instrument must be brief, easy to administer, and valid. In particular, where validity is concerned, the instrument must be able to determine whether the children ($\geq$ 24 months of age) and women served by WIC are meeting the quantitative recommendation for physical activity outlined in the *Dietary Guidelines*. Furthermore, the instrument must be valid across the different populations served by WIC (e.g., rural and urban or African American and white).

Women

Although there are several physical activity questionnaires for adults that have undergone extensive validity testing (Sallis and Saelens, 2000), the staff or client burden of most questionnaires is too great to meet the operational constraints of WIC. This is mainly because of the time involved in capturing all the characteristics of specific physical activity behaviors (i.e., type, frequency, duration, and intensity of each activity) that are necessary for a valid physical activity assessment of an individual. Furthermore, in physical activity assessment, it is even less clear than in diet assessment what reporting period (past day, week, or month) is required to reliably assess habitual activity levels of an individual (Baranowski and de Moor, 2000; Trost et al., 2000). Thus, the cognitive demands of recalling the performance of varied activities over time, while also including the dimensions of frequency, duration, and intensity, is likely to make the valid classification of any individual's physical activity an unachievable goal, regardless of that individual's available time or educational level.

Complicating physical activity assessment is the fact that the *Dietary Guidelines* emphasize moderate, as opposed to vigorous, physical activity. This emphasis arises appropriately from the evidence of the health benefits of moderate levels of physical activity (HHS, 1996). However, the level of moderate activity, as compared to vigorous activity, is far more difficult to determine for an individual because individuals differ greatly in their perceptions of what constitutes moderate activity and in their memory of that activity (Baranowski et al., 1992).

For the target adult population served by WIC, low-income women who are pregnant and/or who are caring for infants and preschool children, a large amount of physical activity may come from housework, childcare activities, occupational activity, or walking for transportation (rather than as a leisure-time activity). To the extent that a physical activity assessment tool does not adequately characterize these moderate activities, the levels of physical activity in WIC women may be greatly underestimated (Ainsworth, 2000a, 2000b; Ainsworth et al., 1999).

In summary, there are no currently available instruments for assessing physical activity in adults that meet the operational constraints of WIC and that can also accurately assess whether an individual is meeting the quantitative physical activity guideline in the *Dietary Guidelines*. Limitations in human cognition make it unlikely that an instrument could ever be developed that would accurately classify an individual's physical activity level for purposes of WIC certification. As with diet recall, accurately recalling and characterizing the varied behaviors that constitute an individual's physical activity level is too complex for the human mind.

Children

The cognitive limitations of preschool children require a parent or other adult caretaker to report on a child's physical activity. Thus, the physical activity instruments used for children are more properly referred to as "parent" or "caretaker" reports than as "self" reports. The two available instruments in which an adult reports on the child's activity were included as part of a recent comprehensive review of self-report instruments for assessing physical activity (Sallis and Saelens, 2000). Both instruments used logs or diaries rather than recalls of the child's activity (Harro, 1997; Manios et al., 1998). Furthermore, only one study (Harro, 1997) involved 4- and 5-year-olds, and neither involved children younger than 4 years of age. Thus, there are no published activity recall instruments for preschool children that could be evaluated by the committee for assessing the physical activity guideline for children that is provided in the *Dietary Guidelines*.

CONCLUSIONS REGARDING THE ROLE OF PHYSICAL ACTIVITY ASSESSMENT FOR ELIGIBILITY DETERMINATION

The committee concludes that there are not now, nor will there likely ever be, valid physical activity assessment tools that can distinguish ineligible individuals from eligible individuals for WIC based on their physical activity levels. Thus, failure to meet the recommend levels of physical activity in the *Dietary Guidelines* should *not* be used to determine eligibility of individuals for WIC services.

However, as with assessment of food intake, there are still at least two possible roles of physical activity assessment in WIC. These roles would help support WIC's mission in the primary prevention of nutrition-related chronic disease, especially the prevention of overweight and obesity. One role of physical activity assessment would be to aid in education and counseling. A second role would be in monitoring groups of individuals or target populations within WIC who may be at higher risk for low physical activity levels and/or who may benefit most from interventions within WIC to increase physical activity levels.

Physical activity assessment tools may be valid for assessing physical activity levels within groups even if they are not valid for assessing individuals. This is primarily due to the high levels of day-to-day variability in physical activity and other reporting errors that greatly affect the validity of assessing physical activity levels in individuals, but do not as greatly affect assessing physical activity levels in groups. Even if valid tools for group assessment were developed in the future, for these tools to be feasible for use in WIC, they would still need to be evaluated in terms of the other criteria within the committee's framework (see Chapter 4). For example, a valid physical activity assessment tool would also need to be brief and easy to administer.

For preschool children, the committee did not identify a physical activity recall instrument even under development. For women in WIC, perhaps, the most promising tools for group assessment of physical activity are the physical activity modules used in the Centers for Disease Control and Prevention's Behavioral Risk Factor Surveillance System (BRFSS) (Macera and Pratt, 2000; Troiano et al., 2001; Washburn et al., 2000). In the 2000 BRFSS, there is an 11-item physical activity module with the items in various domains as follows: occupation, 1 item; walking, 3 items; moderate physical activity, 3 items; vigorous physical activity, 3 items; and strength and flexibility, 1 item. Furthermore, there is also a very brief 3-item module now under development (moderate physical activity, 2 items; vigorous physical activity, 1 item) (CDC, 2001). In the development of this brief 3-item module, the questions have undergone cognitive interviewing and subsequent revision based on that interviewing. After these revisions, the questions will be validated in a number of populations against other measures of physical activity and energy expenditure.

While this research process may hold some promise for the development of a useful tool to assess physical activity levels at the group level among women in WIC, the tool will not produce valid measures for determining individual eligibility. It is impossible for three questions to accurately assess an individual's activity by capturing information about frequency, self-perceived intensity, and duration of activity within a reference period. The correlations between these questions and direct measures of physical activity are unlikely to be greater than 0.4, given the prior work in this area (Ainsworth et al., 1993a; Kriska and Caspersen, 1997). However, these correlations may be adequate for assessment at the group level. Thus, this 3-item module may hold the most promise for WIC because of (1) the extensive effort being placed on its development, including testing in a variety of populations, (2) its brevity, and (3) its ability to classify groups in terms of meeting the quantitative physical activity guideline with the *Dietary Guidelines*. Additionally, these modules would allow WIC to determine whether groups of enrolled women are meeting the physical activity targets outlined in *Healthy People 2010* (HHS, 2000).

RECOMMENDATIONS FOR FUTURE RESEARCH

The principal target groups within WIC for increasing physical activity are children 2 to 5 years of age, and pregnant and postpartum women. As indicated previously, physical activity assessment in WIC, like diet assessment, will have utility only at the group level. This is because even adult women, regardless of their educational level, can not accurately recall their own or their children's physical activity. Such group assessments, however, are still important for education and monitoring, as described above, and research is required to overcome some of the challenges that exist in the valid, group-level assessment of physical activity in those served by WIC.

Several methods of assessing physical activity that are used in research (e.g., activity diaries or logs, direct observation of activity, motion sensors and heart rate monitoring [Baranowski et al., 1992; Goran, 1998; Kohl et al., 2000; Kriska and Caspersen, 1997; Pate, 1993; Sallis and Saelens, 2000; Welk et al., 2000]) could be used as "gold standard" references to conduct validity and reliability studies of practical instruments for WIC to assess physical activity at the group level using recalls. For example, such research might compare the results of a physical activity recall questionnaire (completed by the mother for her preschool child) against data from motion sensors that assess acceleration of the child's body in three dimensions (Freedson and Miller, 2000).

Beyond the significant challenge of adequately describing physical activity levels in the WIC population, little is known about the factors influencing physical activity in the WIC population. It is widely perceived, for example, that concern about neighborhood safety is a major barrier to physical activity. However, the research base supporting this notion is small, and little is known about the factors that, if modified, could improve perceptions abut neighborhood safety, and thereby possibly increase physical activity levels. Whether preschool children or their mothers will be more active if they spend more time outdoors or less time watching television is not known.

However, the research to identify potential target indicators of physical activity must come after efforts to improve physical activity assessment, because target indicators cannot be identified without valid physical activity assessment tools. Furthermore, once behavioral targets are identified, interventions to modify these intermediate targets cannot be assessed without some measure of physical activity, which is the ultimate target of change.

7

Behavioral Indicators of Diet and Physical Activity

Chapters 5 and 6 attempted to show that, for the purpose of determining eligibility for WIC services, one cannot make a valid and reliable assessment of an individual's diet or physical activity patterns using conventional diet and activity assessment tools. For this reason in part, it has been suggested that there may be alternative practical measures that are strongly correlated with diet and activity that could be used in determining eligibility for WIC services. One such method would be the use of behavioral indicators. This chapter explores the concept of behavioral indicators and their possible role in the assessment of an individual's dietary and physical activity patterns for the purposes of determining *failure to meet Dietary Guidelines* and therefore WIC eligibility.

Despite the theoretical and practical attractiveness of a behavioral model for dietary risk assessment, only limited research has been conducted to confirm the relationships among behavioral variables, dietary adequacy or appropriateness, nutrient intake, and health outcomes. There is no one instrument with demonstrated validity and reliability that assesses the many behavioral aspects of diet. In most cases in the literature, these practices or patterns were collected as an adjunct to or coded from other more lengthy dietary assessment methods.

Taken together, the *Dietary Guidelines*, the current WIC eligibility criteria, and the charge of the committee place more emphasis on diet than on activity. Accordingly, this review of behavioral indicators focuses more on diet than on activity. After reviewing the literature on behavioral indicators of diet, this chapter concludes with brief examples of how behavioral indicators might also apply to physical activity assessment, and it provides a more detailed review of one important potential indicator of activity—television viewing.

THE CONCEPT OF BEHAVIORAL INDICATORS

As previously discussed, diet and physical activity are both extremely complex behaviors expressed as systematic patterns that are the end result of a complex series of many decisions (Baranowski, 1997b; Campbell and Desjardins, 1989). These decisions are affected by contextual factors that can be considered behavioral indicators, in that these indicators influence or reflect diet or activity but do not attempt to directly measure diet or activity. For example, many contextual factors affect a person's diet, such as where one eats; who else is present and why; the cost, convenience, or familiarity of certain foods; and the presence of emotional states, such as loneliness or boredom, that can serve as eating cues. Similarly, activity levels can also be affected by contextual factors like the weather, the availability of safe outdoor areas, the support or interest of family and peers, and the presence of competing sedentary activities such as television viewing. Interest in using these behavioral indicators in WIC may also be increased by the untested assumption that, in comparison to conventional tools for assessing diet and activity, these indicators may be easier to recall, less susceptible to various types of reporting bias, and therefore most appropriate targets for behavioral counseling.

A distinction can be drawn between *surrogate* and *target* behavioral indicators (See Box 7-1). Surrogate indicators are those that can be used in place of usual dietary or physical activity assessment procedures. For example, the *frequency of eating a meal as a family* is a possible surrogate indicator because it has been shown that families who eat dinner together tend to eat better diets (Gillman et al., 2000). If the frequency of eating family meals could be assessed more reliably than what foods a person usually eats, and if family meal eating

---

BOX 7-1 Definitions of Two Behavioral Indicators

Surrogate Behavioral Indicators
• indicators that are correlated with one or more aspects of diet or activity and could be used to measure those aspects of diet or activity

Target Behavioral Indicators
• indicators that determine one or more aspects of diet or activity and, if changed, would result in changes in diet or activity

> **BOX 7-2** Criteria for Establishing Surrogate or Target Behavioral Indicators
>
> Surrogate Behavioral Criteria
> - behavior is substantially correlated with some aspect of diet or activity
> - behavior is consistently correlated with some aspect of diet or activity
> - behavior is more reliably assessed than corresponding aspect of diet or activity
>
> Target Behavioral Criteria
> - behavioral indicator causes some aspect of diet or activity
> - behavioral indicator is modifiable
> - changes in the behavioral indicator result in substantial change in the diet or activity

could consistently and substantially discriminate between the higher consumption of certain foods (e.g., fruit and vegetables) and lower consumption of other foods (e.g., low nutrient-dense foods), then assessment of *frequency of eating a meal as a family* could be used as a surrogate for assessment of actual food intake when determining dietary risk (see Box 7-2). In evaluating the potential of using surrogate indicators for the purposes of determining WIC eligibility, one important issue is the level of reliability and validity of these surrogate measures in comparison to the conventional food-based assessment procedures such as dietary recalls. If the validity and reliability of the surrogate indicators are not higher than those for food-based assessment procedures, then there is little advantage to using the surrogate. If the surrogate is not substantially correlated with true consumption, then misclassification error increases substantially.

Target indicators are those that identify precursors of diet or activity, which, if changed, result in improved dietary intake or levels of physical activity (Nicklas et al., in press; Siega-Riz et al., 2000). If behavioral indicators are causative of the diet or activity patterns, the behaviors are modifiable, and if the changes result in improved diet or activity practices, then they could be targets for WIC-related nutrition education efforts (see Box 7-2). To continue with the prior example, if families could be easily encouraged to more frequently eat meals together, and increased family dinners resulted in improved dietary intake, then *frequency of eating a meal as a family* is a likely target indicator for change.

The key issue in selecting a target indicator is whether the behavioral indicator is modifiable and whether a change in the indicator results in a change in diet or activity. If a change in the target indicator is possible but is not substantially related to an alteration in diet or activity, then there would be little reason to attempt to change the target indicator. Virtually any correlate of diet or activity behavior can be considered for status as a surrogate or target, but must be demonstrated to meet the corresponding criteria for such status (see Box 7-2).

BEHAVIORAL INDICATORS OF DIET

Categories of Behavioral Indicators of Diet

This literature review attempts to identify a variety of examples of behavioral diet indicators that may be considered for surrogate or target indicators for use in the WIC program. Possible surrogate or target behavioral practices were each placed within one of the following categories: indicator foods; food, eating, or dietary patterns; meal patterns; health-related behaviors; psychosocial characteristics; parent food practices; ecological factors; or alternative technology. Most of the research on behaviors as possible surrogates for measures of dietary intake was not conducted with the intent of validating surrogates. Rather, it was conducted within the framework of understanding correlates of dietary intake. There are not many such studies. All of the methods used as indicators of validity for this purpose were self-reported (subjective), including food records. Table 7-1 summarizes the categories and provides the range of validity and reliability coefficients. Table 7-2 provides examples of indicators for each category as well as the references in which the indicator was studied.

Indicator foods are single foods, consumed either for specific meals (e.g., eggs for breakfast) or during the day as a whole (e.g., red meat), that are related to variations in dietary intake usually in regard to nutrients (e.g., eat more total calories). Since indicator foods reflect rather than determine diet, they have potential as surrogate, but not target, indicators.

Food, eating, or dietary patterns are either groups of foods commonly eaten together (usually based on a statistical procedure called factor analysis), or groups of people who commonly eat certain types of food (usually based on a statistical procedure called cluster analysis), or from logically placing practices together related to a particular nutrient (e.g., dietary fat). Since these patterns reflect rather than determine diet, they have primary interest as surrogate indicators.

Meal patterns describe some aspect of an individual's meal behavior other than consumption of specific foods or categories of foods. An example of a meal pattern would be "not eating breakfast." Meal patterns could be surrogate or target behavior indicators, depending on whether the practice determines the dietary intake of interest.

Health-related behavior concerns the assessment of other behaviors related to health. For example, smoking is correlated with one or most aspects of dietary

TABLE 7-1 Categories of Behavioral Indicators of Diet

Behavioral Indicator	Range of Reliability Coefficients	Range of Validity Coefficients
Indicator foods		
Consumption of specific foods (either at a specific meal or for the day as a whole)	Not reported	Not reported
Food, eating, or dietary patterns	Most none	Substantial relationships between factors and consumption
Groups of foods or categories of foods that are usually consumed or practiced together	$\alpha = 0.54$–0.76 trt $= 0.67$–0.90	Partial correlation $r = -0.29$ to -0.68 from 0.10 to 0.39
Meal patterns		
Differences in meal or snack consumption	Not reported	Partial $r \leq 0.10$
Health-related behaviors		
Some other health-related behavior	Not reported	Not reported
Psychosocial characteristics		
Psychosocial variables related to food intake Clusters of such variables	From < 0.10 to > 0.90	Most are ≤ 0.30
Parent food practices		
Parent behavior in regard to some aspect of child's dietary behavior	From < 0.10 to > 0.90	Most are ≤ 0.30
Ecological factors		
Aspects of the home or neighborhood	From < 0.5 to 0.9 for some indicators	More are ≤ 0.30

intake. It appears that health-related behaviors reflect, rather than cause, dietary behavior and thereby have more potential as surrogate indicators.

Certain *psychosocial characteristics,* such as food preferences or self-efficacy related to altering diet, have been related to dietary intake. Likewise, aggregates or clusters of these psychosocial characteristics have also been shown to correlate with dietary intake in marketing studies. Although the causal status of these psychosocial characteristics has not been clearly demonstrated, if established, they could become target indicators.

TABLE 7-2 References for Data Bearing on Behavioral Nutrition Indicators by WIC Target Group and Category of Indicator

Practices	25–48 months	Children/Adolescents
Indicator foods		
Eating eggs for breakfast	—	—
Eating ready-to-eat cereal for breakfast	—	Nicklas et al., in press
Eating coffee, soft drink, or dessert alone for breakfast	—	—
Added sugar	—	Forshee and Storey, 2001
Milk consumption	—	Ballew et al., 2000
Juice consumption	—	Ballew et al., 2000
Soft drink consumption	—	Ballew et al., 2000
Food, eating, or dietary patterns		
Many factors	—	—
Prudent diet factor	—	—
Western diet factor	—	—
Fat practices	—	—
Many clusters	—	—
Dietary adequacy	—	—
Vegetarian	—	Jacobs and Dwyer, 1988
Meal patterns		
Meal consistency	—	Siega-Riz et al., 1998
Regularly eat breakfast	—	Sampson et al., 1995
Snacking	—	—
Eating out of home frequently	—	—
Eating fast food frequently	—	—
Eating span	—	Berenson et al., 1980
Longest fast > 13 hours	—	—
Related behaviors (self)		
Smoking	—	—
Physical activity	—	Rosmond et al., 2000
Eating while watching television	—	Coon et al., 2001

Pregnant	Lactating	Postpartum	Adults
—	—	—	Siega-Riz et al., 2000
—	—	—	Siega-Riz et al., 2000
—	—	—	Siega-Riz et al., 2000
—	—	—	—
—	—	—	—
—	—	—	—
—	—	—	—
—	—	—	Randall et al., 1990, 1991b; Wolff and Wolff, 1995
—	—	—	Fung et al., 2001
—	—	—	Fung et al., 2001
—	—	—	Kristal et al., 1990
—	—	—	Huijbregts et al., 1995; Millen et al., 2001; Slattery et al., 1998; Wirfalt and Jeffery, 1997
—	—	—	Knol and Haughton, 1998
—	—	—	Donovan and Gibson, 1996; Janelle and Barr, 1995
—	—	—	—
—	—	—	Nicklas et al., 1998; Siega-Riz et al., 2000
—	—	—	Zizza et al., 2001
—	—	—	Clemens et al., 1999; McCrory et al., 1999
—	—	—	French et al., 2000
—	—	—	—
—	—	—	—
Haste et al., 1990	—	—	Huijbregts et al., 1995; Ma et al., 2000; Randall et al., 1991a; Tucker et al., 1992
—	—	—	Matthews et al., 1997; Rogers et al., 1995; Slattery et al., 1998
—	—	—	—

continued

TABLE 7-2 Continued

Practices	25–48 months	Children/Adolescents
Psychosocial characteristics and clusters		
Psychosocial variables	—	Baranowski et al., 1999
Psychosocial clusters	—	—
Parent food practices	—	Baranowski, 1997a; Nicklas et al., 2001
Ecological factors		
Availability of whole fruit, 100% juice, and vegetable (FJV) at home	—	Hearn et al., 1998; Kratt et al., 2000
Availability of FJV in local restaurants	—	Edmonds et al., 2001
Socioeconomic status	—	—
Household food insecurity	—	—

Parent food practices concern parent behaviors in regard to their child's food consumption (e.g., an authoritative parenting style in which both emotional support and limit-seeking occur together). Parent food practices could be responses to child food behavior or could be causative. If shown to be causative, they could be surrogate or target indicators.

Ecological factors are aspects of the family or home environment related to food intake (e.g., home availability or accessibility of certain foods). If ecological factors are demonstrated to be causative of dietary behavior, they could become surrogate or target indicators.

Review of Literature on Behavioral Indicators of Diet

Published studies on behavioral indicators of diet in WIC target groups are very limited. While studies on correlates of diet have been conducted with children older than 5 years of age, there are very few addressing children under 5 years. In addition, much of the work on correlates of diet in adults has occurred among adults in general, not usually among adults in the WIC targeted categories (see Table 7-2). For this reason, the following literature review will cover children older than those served by WIC and covers women in general rather than low-income women specifically.

Since many of these behavioral indicators of diet have been abstracted from other assessment instruments (e.g., 24-hour dietary recalls, food frequency questionnaires), few indicators of reliability have been reported in the literature. Additionally, very few estimates of the strength of relationships of these

Pregnant	Lactating	Postpartum	Adults
—	—	—	Baranowski et al., 1999
—	—	—	Dutta and Youn, 1999; Glanz et al., 1998
—	—	—	Baranowski, 1997a; Nicklas et al., 2001
—	—	—	—
—	—	—	—
—	—	—	Haste et al., 1990; Hupkens et al., 1997
—	—	—	Casey et al., 2001; Derrickson et al., 2001; Lee and Fongillo, 2001; Tarasuk and Beaton, 1999

indicators with diet have been reported, and those that have been reported used different indicators of strength (e.g., correlation coefficients, F test values). Thus, no attempt was made to systematically report reliability coefficients or the strengths of relationships.

Indicator Foods

Indicator foods have been used to understand variations in what people eat. In general, consumption of an indicator food has been associated with intakes of nutrients, food groups, or energy. Thus, briefly assessing consumption of an indicator food could provide an index of consumption of a WIC nutrient or food group. For example, data from 24-hour recalls from a nationally representative sample of adults in the 1994–1996 Continuing Survey of Food Intakes by Individuals (CSFII) (n = 15,641) indicated that adults ate the following selected breakfast items: eggs (15 percent); ready-to-eat cereal (17 percent); bread only (22 percent); cooked cereal (4 percent); fruit only (6 percent); coffee, soft drink, and/or high-fat dessert (15 percent); or other (3 percent) (Siega-Riz et al., 2000). Those eating an egg-based breakfast consumed more total calories and had a higher percentage of calories from fat for breakfast, but lower carbohydrates, calcium, folate, and iron. Those consuming coffee, soft drink, and/or dessert consumed the fewest breakfast calories, lower daily intakes of protein, fiber, and folate, and the highest intake of saturated fat (Siega-Riz et al., 2000). The consumption of ready-to-eat cereal for breakfast was associated with consumption of lower total fat, and more folic acid, iron, niacin, vitamin A, vitamin C, and zinc per dollar spent than those who ate fast food or other breakfasts (Nicklas et al., in press).

Combining all children (> 2 years old) and adults in the 1994–1996 CSFII data set, and after controlling for age, gender, and consumption of other macronutrients, people who ate more added sugar also tended to consume more grains and lean meat, but less vegetables, fruit, and dairy, and more vitamin C and iron, but less vitamin A, calcium, and folate (Forshee and Storey, 2001). These relationships varied, however, among children by age of the child from 6 to 11 years versus 12 to 19 years. All relationships were weak.

Children in the CSFII data set who drank more milk were more likely to have significantly higher intakes of vitamin A, folate, vitamin B_{12}, calcium, and magnesium (in all age groups: 2–5 years, 6–11 years, and 12–17 years). Similarly, children in all age groups who drank more 100 percent juice were more likely to consume more vitamin C and folate (Forshee and Storey, 2001). However, children who drank more 100 percent juice were less likely to consume vitamin B_{12} among 12- to 17-year-olds, but not among other age groups. Children who drank more carbonated beverages were significantly less likely to consume vitamin A among all age groups. In those 2 to 11 years old, but not those 12 to 17 years old, carbonated beverage drinkers had lower vitamin C and calcium intakes (Ballew et al., 2000). For all age groups, children who drank more carbonated beverages were less likely to consume milk and 100 percent fruit juice (Ballew et al., 2000).

Food, Eating, or Dietary Patterns

Food, eating, or dietary patterns are consistent groupings of foods, usually determined by statistical techniques. Using food frequency data from 2,255 adults in the Western New York Diet Study (1975–1986), Randall and colleagues (1991b) demonstrated substantial intercorrelations in consumption among food groups and nutrients. Using the same data set, they reported a principal components analysis across 110 foods. Also called factor analysis, this technique identifies common patterns in foods consumed. Nine factors were extracted, which they interpreted as (1) salad, (2) Southern European/healthful, (3) fruit, (4) low cost, (5) dessert, (6) staple vegetables, (7) costly, (8) health foods, and (9) nonuse (Randall et al., 1990). Each factor was significantly correlated with several key macro- and micronutrients (e.g., energy, dietary fat, dietary fiber, and vitamins A and C). Some differences in factor structures were determined between males and females (Randall et al., 1991b). These factors correlated in expected directions with National Cancer Institute-specified consumption of dietary fat; dietary fiber density; vegetable diversity; fruit diversity; alcoholic beverage; cured, pickled, and smoked meats and fish and charbroiled meat and poultry; and sodium (Randall et al., 1991b). Using tertiles on the factor scores, some of these relationships appeared to be strong, for example, high fat factor with dietary fat (F = 183.1); fruit factor with dietary fiber density (F = 108.4); salad factor (F = 262.4), healthful factor (F = 357.6), and traditional factor (F = 206.3) with vegetable diversity; fruit factor with fruit diversity (F = 758.8); and high fat factor with total alcohol consumption (F = 133.3) (Randall et al., 1991b).

Using food frequency questionnaires (FFQs) from the Hispanic Health and Nutrition Examination Survey (Hispanic HANES), eating patterns were identified using factor analysis in 49 Mexican-American mothers (Wolff and Wolff, 1995). Seven eating pattern factors were extracted: nutrient-dense, traditional, transitional, nutrient-dilute, protein-rich, high-fat dairy, and mixed dishes. After controlling for demographic and related variables, the nutrient-dense (fruit, vegetables, low-fat dairy) and protein-rich eating patterns were associated with increased birth weight, while the transitional eating pattern was associated with decreased birth weight (Wolff and Wolff, 1995). The relationships, however, were weak.

Based on the anthropological theory of core foods, an 18-item questionnaire was developed to assess aspects of reduced dietary fat practices (Kristal et al., 1990). A confirmatory factor analysis of these items revealed five factors: (1) avoiding fat as a seasoning, (2) avoiding meat, (3) modifying high fat foods, (4) substituting high-fat foods with specially manufactured low-fat foods, and (5) replacing high-fat foods with low-fat alternatives (Kristal et al., 1990). The five scales had modest Cronbach alpha reliabilities (α = 0.54–0.76) and higher test–retest reliabilities (trt = 0.67–0.90). The validity correlations with percent energy as fat varied from -0.29 to -0.68 (Kristal et al., 1990). At least one study found that variables from such food behavior questions correlated with breast cancer rates, while nutrients from FFQs did not (Byrne et al., 1996).

Other investigators have employed cluster analysis as a statistical technique for identifying dietary patterns. Cluster analysis groups people into relatively homogeneous categories of consumption. One group found four cluster-determined dietary groups among noninstitutionalized senior citizens: (1) alcohol, (2) milk, cereals, and fruit, (3) bread and poultry, and (4) meat and potatoes (Tucker et al., 1992). Those in the milk, cereal, and fruit cluster had the highest intake of micronutrients and the best hematologic profile. Those in the meat and potatoes cluster had the lowest intake of micronutrients, while those in the bread and poultry cluster had the lowest reported energy intake, but the highest body mass index (BMI) (Tucker et al., 1992). Pooling FFQ data from three studies conducted with adults in the upper Midwest, six food cluster groups were determined: (1) high intake of soft drinks, (2) high intake of pastries, (3) high intake of skim milk, (4) high intake of meat, (5) high intake of meat and cheese, and (6) high intake of white bread (Wirfalt and Jeffery, 1997). Participants in the high soft drink consumption cluster had low intake of protein, fiber, and calcium and higher BMI among men, but not women. Those in the high meat and high pastry clusters had higher dietary fat intake (Wirfalt and Jeffery, 1997).

As part of the Framingham Offspring-Spouse study of 1,828 adult women, five eating pattern clusters were determined: (1) heart healthy, (2) light eating, (3) wine and moderate eating, (4) high-fat, and (5) empty calories (Millen et al., 2001). Statistically significant differences across eating patterns were detected for a broad variety of macro- and micronutrients and cardiovascular disease risk factors. Some of these relationships were strong, but most were not (Millen et al., 2001).

One dietary pattern cluster that is easy to recognize is vegetarianism. There are several forms of vegetarianism (e.g., vegans use no animal products, lacto-vegetarians use milk products in addition to plant products, lacto-ovo-vegetarians use milk and egg products in addition to plant products, and various more restrictive practices [Jacobs and Dwyer, 1988]) that potentially could be easily identified through one self-report question. Among women in western Canada with better health practices in general, vegetarians tended to have lower BMI, and especially lower percent body fat (Janelle and Barr, 1995). Among female adolescents in southern Ontario, there were no statistically significant differences in energy consumed across lacto-ovo-vegetarians, semi-vegetarians, and omnivorous groups (Donovan and Gibson, 1996). Lacto-ovo-vegetarians tended to consume less protein and niacin, but more dietary fiber, copper, and manganese than omnivorous groups, but these differences were small. Semi-vegetarians had the greatest risk of inadequate calorie, protein, iron, zinc, and vitamin C intake (Donovan and Gibson, 1996).

Food Patterns

Food patterns were developed to identify naturally occurring groupings in foods consumed. Interest in food patterns has arisen, in part, because data on the intake of single nutrients are very limited in their ability to predict the development of those chronic diseases that are suspected to be related to diet (Jacques and Tucker, 2001). Food patterns related to health issues of concern to WIC (e.g., obesity) may provide important targets because they are the foods of interest. Because they would be dependent on tools similar to FFQs, it appears unlikely that food patterns could be valid or reliable enough to be used for eligibility determination.

Meal Patterns

Meal patterns characterize aspects of meals such as whether specific meals or snacks were consumed, where the meals were consumed, or over what time period during the day one ate. For example, assessing whether a child consistently ate breakfast could be an easy way to assess total caloric intake.

Using three 24-hour diet recalls from the 1989–1999 CSFII, meal patterns were analyzed among a nationally representative sample of 1,310 adolescents (11–18 years of age) (Siega-Riz et al., 1998). On any one day, about 58 percent of adolescents ate three meals plus snacks. The second most common meal pattern was breakfast, dinner, and snacks (about 15 percent). About 3 percent ate only one meal or only snacks on any particular day. Adolescents were categorized into consistent, moderately consistent, and inconsistent meal patterns based on how many meals were consumed across the 3 days of assessment. Adolescents with consistent meal plans ate more total calories, fiber, calcium, iron, vitamin E, fruit and vegetable servings, grain and legume servings, and sodium, but had a lower diet quality index (Siega-Riz et al., 1998).

Skipping Breakfast. Whether a person skipped breakfast or not could be assessed by a single question. In the 1994–1996 CSFII data with a nationally representative sample of 15,641 adults, 17 percent did not consume breakfast, but this percentage was higher in 18- to 40-year-olds (23 percent) than in 41- to 65-year-olds (13 percent) (Siega-Riz et al., 2000). Among 509 young adults in Bogalusa, Louisiana (studied from 1988–1991), using 24-hour diet recalls, 37 percent skipped breakfast the previous day (Nicklas et al., 1998). Those not eating breakfast consumed 568 fewer calories per day, less protein, less saturated fat, but 121 mg more cholesterol. Men who skipped breakfast consumed less total fat than all females or males eating breakfast (Nicklas et al., 1998). Those not eating breakfast were less likely to consume two-thirds or more of the Recommended Dietary Allowance (RDA) for a variety of micronutrients, but even among those eating breakfast, those achieving two-thirds or more of the RDA varied from approximately 40 to 90 percent (Nicklas et al., 1998). Among 1,151 mostly lower-income African-American second to fifth grade children in New Jersey who completed a 24-hour diet recall and 4 days of food surveys (Sampson et al., 1995), children not eating breakfast before school varied from 22 to 26 percent per day. Across all 4 days, 71 percent reported eating breakfast each day and 4 percent reported eating breakfast for none of the days, with no differences by gender. Children who skipped breakfast had significantly lower daily intakes of calories and micronutrients. While those who skipped breakfast consumed a higher percentage of calories from fat, they had lower intakes of cholesterol and sodium. There was no difference between groups in BMI (Sampson et al., 1995).

Snacking Patterns. Using 24-hour diet recall data from three CSFII data sets (1977–1978, 1989–1991, 1994–1996), snacking patterns were assessed in nationally representative samples of young adults (19–29 years of age) (Zizza et al., 2001). The percentage of young adults who did not snack across the multiple days of assessment changed from 23.4, to 25.8, to 15.6 percent across the three time intervals. The average number of snacking occasions per day increased from 1.70, to 1.69, to 1.92. The calories consumed per snacking occasion increased from 247, to 265, to 313. This increase in calories was accounted for in part by the caloric density per gram of snack food, which increased from 1.05, to 1.30, to 1.32. The caloric density per gram of food at meals remained a near constant 1.11 to 1.13 across the three time intervals. In each year, those who snacked consumed more energy, more carbohydrates (but not as a percentage of calories), more fat (but not as a percentage of calories), and more saturated fat (Zizza et al., 2001).

Meals Away from Home. Using a 7-day food record from 129 young women (average age 30 years), the sample was divided into more frequent events (6–13 times per week), or less frequent events (≤ 5 times per week) of eating meals outside the home (Clemens et al., 1999). Women who ate out more frequently consumed more total calories, fat, carbohydrates, protein, and sodium, but not fiber or calcium.

Using an FFQ with 73 healthy men and women, there was substantial variability in the rate of eating outside the home: 7.5 ± 8.5 times per month (McCrory et al., 1999). After statistically controlling for demographic variables, people who ate outside the home more frequently had higher BMIs ($r = 0.36$). After also controlling for amount of physical activity, the relationship increased ($r = 0.42$). People who ate outside the home more frequently consumed more energy ($r = 0.59$), more dietary fat ($r = 0.28$), and less fiber ($r = -0.45$) (McCrory et al., 1999).

Focusing more specifically on fast food consumption, FFQs were given to 891 women (20 to 45 years of age) enrolled in a weight gain prevention study. Results indicated that 21 percent of the women had three or more fast food-eating events in a week. Additionally, 16 percent reported two events, 39 percent reported one event, and 24 percent reported none (French et al., 2000). Women who reported the highest number of fast food-eating events (highest tertile or $X = 3.3$ events) consumed significantly more total calories, fat as a percentage of calories, hamburgers, french fries, and soft drinks. Additionally they consumed less dietary fiber, vegetables, and fruit (French et al., 2000). Women who increased the frequency of eating out over 3 years consumed more total calories, percent of energy as fat, hamburgers, french fries, and soft drinks, and less vegetables. Weight increased with increased fast food consumption (French et al., 2000).

Eating Span. Using 24-hour diet recalls among 10-year-old children in the Bogalusa study, eating span was defined as the number of hours from first food or beverage consumed to last consumed (Berenson et al., 1980). Three groups were identified: short span (10 hours or less, $n = 19$); moderate span (10 to 13 hours, $n = 95$), and long span (13 hours or more, $n = 71$). There were no gender differences in span. Children with a longer eating span consistently consumed 40 percent more than short span and 20 percent more than moderate span children of calories, protein, fat, carbohydrate, and sodium. Children with the longer eating span also had higher total serum cholesterol (Berenson et al., 1980).

Pregnant women who regularly fasted more than 13 hours (overnight) were more likely to have premature and small-for-gestational-growth babies (Siega-Riz et al., 2000). Although this should be a relatively easily measured phenomenon, little has been published about it or its measurement. There are likely other behavioral phenomena that have similar health implications. While research needs to identify the physiological and behavioral processes that account for this adverse outcome, behavior change programs can be initiated to attempt to change these fasting patterns and in turn assess the extent to which change in the fasting pattern results in improved pregnancy outcome.

Related Health Behaviors

Research has revealed that there are patterns across several health behaviors. For example, people who smoke have less healthy diets (Ma et al., 2000). Since regular smoking can be relatively easily assessed, it is possible that this could provide important surrogate or target behavioral indicators. Among the previously described dietary pattern studies using FFQs, smoking was negatively correlated with the salad, fruit, healthful, and whole grain factors, and positively correlated with the high-fat factor among men, and with similar patterns among women (Randall et al., 1991a). Nonsmokers were more common in the healthy diet cluster even after controlling for possible confounders (Huijbregts et al., 1995). Smoking was most common in the alcohol cluster (Tucker et al., 1992).

Using two 24-hour diet recalls in the 1994–1996 CSFII, whether a person smoked (current, former, or non) or drank alcohol (abstainers, occasional, moderate, or liberal drinkers) were assessed among a nationally representative sample of 6,745 adults (19 years of age and older) (Ma et al., 2000). The smoking and drinking subgroups differed in age, income, education, BMI, exercise, and other behavior, which could confound other relationships. Current and former smokers drank more alcohol than nonsmokers. Men and women who smoked the most cigarettes reported the lowest consumption of fruit, carotenes, and vitamin C. Men and women who drank the most alcohol reported the lowest consumption of fruit; grain; carbohydrates, fat and protein as a percent of calories; carotenes; and dietary fiber (Ma et al., 2000).

Using a 7-day weighed dietary intake record of women in London at 28 ($n = 206$) and at 36 weeks ($n = 178$) of gestation, intake was compared between smokers (≥ 15 cigarettes per day, $n = 83$) and nonsmokers ($n = 101$) (Haste et al., 1990). Smokers consumed less macro- and micronutrients, whether expressed as nutrients or nutrient density, even after controlling for social class (Haste et al., 1990).

In one of the diet pattern studies described earlier, leisure time physical activity was higher in those consuming a prudent diet (Slattery et al., 1998). Using an FFQ with 211 less well-educated adult patients in the General Medicine Clinic in Syracuse, New York, diet and physical activity were assessed (Rogers et al., 1995). Patients with less physical activity were less likely to consume vegetables, fruit (especially those 20 to 49 years of age), and high-fiber grains (Rogers et al., 1995). Using a 7-day diet recall and one 24-hour diet recall with 919 adults in the WATCH hyperlipidemia trial, physical activity was assessed using a new questionnaire that assessed type, duration, and intensity of regular activity (Matthews et al., 1997). Those reporting more minutes of physical activity reported consuming less fried foods, but there were nonlinear patterns of consumption for other food groups. The nonlinear patterns were also obtained for nutrients consumed (Matthews et al., 1997).

In a randomly selected sample of 40-year-old women ($n = 1,464$) in Sweden, reports of fighting and playing with boys in childhood were positively related, and playing with girl toys and other girls during childhood were negatively related, to the probability of being overweight (Rosmond et al., 2000).

Whether the television was on while 10-year-old children ate breakfast, afternoon snacks, or dinner was assessed in a sample of 91 parent–child pairs, along with three 24-hour diet recalls (Coon et al., 2001). Children for whom the television was on for two or three of the eating occasions consumed less fruit, vegetables, and juice and more meat, pizza, snacks, and carbonated beverages (Coon et al., 2001).

Psychosocial Correlates

A recent review of psychosocial correlates (e.g., self efficacy or preference) of intake of dietary fat, fruit, juice, and vegetables revealed a large body of research employing many different psychosocial constructs. However, most of these relationships were weak to moderate (Baranowski et al., 1999). As a result, there appears to be no advantage to using these as surrogate diet indicators. Alternatively, psychosocial variables have been proposed as the most likely mediators of dietary change interventions (Baranowski et al., 1997, 1998). Thus, better understanding of these relationships may lead to more effective dietary change interventions, which suggests they could be target indicators. A particularly promising avenue of research comes from the realm of social marketing. Market segmentation is a marketing technique that divides the population into relatively homogeneous groups that are related to diet in various ways (Dutta and Youn, 1999; Glanz et al., 1998). The clustering often uses psychosocial variables, and is referred to as "psychographics" (Dutta and Youn, 1999). Thus, empirically identifying profiles of groups of people based on several psychosocial correlates of diet may lead to different, and hopefully more effective, interventions for each group. At the present time, it is not yet clear how one would design interventions using such profiles.

Parent Food Practices

Reviews of family correlates of dietary intake have also appeared recently (Baranowski, 1997a; Nicklas et al., 2001). In a vein similar to the psychosocial variables, the documented relationships have been mostly weak to modest, thereby precluding their use as surrogate diet indicators. Better understanding of these relationships, however, also could suggest improved targets for promoting dietary change in the families of children and in spousal pairs (Baranowski and Hearn, 1997). It appears likely that, since dietary behaviors and practices are established early in life, they have a long-term influence on diet (Baranowski et al., 2000; Costanzo and Woody, 1984). Thus, research on parent food practices as targets for intervention has particular promise for having long-term impacts on the health of both adults and children. (Baranowski et al., 2000).

Ecological or Environmental Correlates

Other possible sources of behavioral indicators of diet are ecological or environmental variables. For example, it could be possible that assessing whether certain foods are available in the home could provide surrogate indicators of consumption of these foods.

Bronfenbrenner (1993) has been a leading advocate of ecological approaches to understanding behavior, but it has only recently been applied to diet behavior (Black, 1999). One decision in the cascade of decisions that result in food consumed at home is what foods are purchased and kept in the home (Baranowski, 1997b; Campbell and Desjardins, 1989), otherwise called availability (e.g., carrots in the refrigerator vegetable bin) (Hearn et al., 1998; Kratt et al., 2000). Accessibility includes whether foods kept in the home are in a form that encourages their consumption at an appropriate time (e.g., clean, scraped, sliced carrots in a plastic bag on a child-accessible shelf next to the child's favorite dip at 3:00 p.m. on a school day). In a large sample of third grade children, whole fruit, 100 percent juice, and vegetable (FJV) availability and accessibility were related to consumption (Hearn et al., 1998). FJV availability and accessibility moderated the relationship of psychosocial variables to consumption (Kratt et al., 2000). School lunch FJV availability was related to child school lunch FJV consumption (Hearn et al., 1998), and availability in restaurants in the same census tract in which participating adolescent males lived was related to adolescent male FJV consumption

(Edmonds et al., 2001). Availability and accessibility were identified as mediators of dietary change in a community intervention project with children (Baranowski et al., in press). A limitation of this research for purposes of behavioral indicators has been the weak relationships obtained ($0.1 \le r \le 0.25$).

A pervasive aspect of the environment is socioeconomic status (SES). In concept, SES indicates the resources available to purchase foods and knowledge of the best foods to buy. In addition, certain values, beliefs, and behaviors may be held in common at different levels of SES. SES is often measured by how much education and/or income a person or family has, and/or their type of occupation. Using the FFQs and an indicator of educational attainment with 849 women from families with school children in three communities in the Netherlands, people at lower levels of SES ate more meat, oils, fats, bread, and potatoes but less cheese, dietary fiber, and vegetables, than other SES levels (Hupkens et al., 1997).

In a health-related behavior study using a 7-day weighed dietary intake and a measure of SES involving coding of occupation of male partner, SES was a significant predictor of consumption of total calories and every macro- and micronutrient (Haste et al., 1990). SES was a significant predictor even after statistically controlling for smoking, which was also shown to be a predictor of consumption of most nutrients (Haste et al., 1990).

One reason low SES may lead to poor diets is the lack of money to purchase food. This has been called "food insufficiency." Using the 1994–1996 CSFII data, when including a single item statement of how often the household did not have enough food to eat in the past 3 months, only 5.9 percent of low-income households (at or below 130 percent of the poverty guideline) reported inadequate food, but 7.9 percent of low-income households with children reported food insufficiency (Casey et al., 2001). No statistically significant differences in nutrient consumption were detected between food-insufficient and food-sufficient, low-income families. Food-insufficient, low-income families consumed fewer servings of dark green leafy vegetables, other vegetables, nuts and seeds, and added sugar, but more eggs, than food-sufficient, low-income families. Only relatively small differences were detected between groups (Casey et al., 2001).

In a sample of 153 women (19–48 years of age) seeking food assistance in Toronto, 15.1 percent reported food insecurity with severe hunger and 35.3 percent reported food insecurity with moderate hunger (Tarasuk and Beaton, 1999). Women reporting food insecurity with severe hunger consumed 1,486 fewer kJ/d than the no food insecurity group and 468 less kJ/d than the food insecure with moderate hunger group. The food insecure with severe hunger group reported lower protein, iron, magnesium, and zinc intake than other groups (Tarasuk and Beaton, 1999).

Evaluation of the Behavioral Indicators of Diet in Relationship to the Suggested Criteria for Dietary Assessment Tools

The committee was asked to consider the possible role of behavior-based indicators in dietary risk assessment. Any candidate behavioral indicator of diet that might be used for the purpose of determining the eligibility of individuals for the WIC program would need to be considered against the eight suggested criteria for evaluating dietary assessment tools described in Chapter 4. In the categories of behavioral indicators of diet that have been reviewed, the committee was unable to identify any indicators that would satisfy the eight evaluation criteria. As with all the food-based, dietary assessment tools, there is a major difficulty with the criteria of reliability and/or validity (criterion 4) for all behavioral indicators where individual assessment is concerned. Indeed, the categories of indicator foods, dietary patterns, and meal patterns are derived from traditional, food-based assessment techniques such as 24-hour dietary recall and FFQs. Furthermore, very little of the research on behavioral indicators has been performed in the populations served by WIC. Finally, there are no randomized trials that attempt to change any target behavioral indicators and measure the impact on diet.

Perhaps a reasonable goal for behavioral measures is to achieve the status of a target indicator and thereby provide a focus for WIC nutrition education. To be a target indicator, the behavioral measure must be demonstrated to correlate with, and be causative of, an important dietary behavior at some reasonably high level; it should be amenable to change through some demonstrated method; and the change in the targeted variable should be demonstrated to be related to changes in the dietary practices of interest. Change in the targeted practice should be relatively easy to accomplish considering the operational constraints of WIC. Although substantial error exists in dietary and behavioral indicator assessment that precludes reasonable accuracy for determining WIC eligibility for individuals, there is merit in doing research on correlates of diet in groups representative of WIC populations. A variety of statistical procedures are available that can correct for known sources of error (Traub, 1994) and thereby provide reasonable tests of relationships. Thus, while a relationship between a behavioral indicator and diet may not be true of any specific individual, it would be true of the group assessed. WIC might then use the findings from such research to make inferences about the behavior of groups (e.g., pregnant Hispanic teenagers) rather than individuals, and to make decisions about the content of dietary counseling that is targeted to the specific groups that have been studied.

BEHAVIORAL INDICATORS OF PHYSICAL ACTIVITY

A literature review has recently been completed on the correlates of physical activity in children (Sallis et al., 2000). While this review did not examine studies in preschool children per se, it did review the literature on correlates in 4- to 12-year-old children. These correlates can all be considered as potential surrogate or target behavioral indicators of physical activity, according to the criteria previously discussed (see Box 7-2). Target indicators, in particular, would be precursors of physical activity. If changed, they would result in increased levels of physical activity and might also serve as the appropriate targets for behavioral counseling efforts.

In the review by Sallis et al., the two strongest correlates with physical activity in children were time spent outdoors (Baranowski et al., 1993; Klesges et al., 1990; Sallis et al., 1993) and access to recreational facilities or play spaces (Garcia et al., 1995; Sallis et al., 1993; Stucky-Ropp and DiLorenzo, 1993). With regard to the factors that parents evaluate in selecting outdoor play spaces for preschoolers, perceived safety may be the most important factor (Sallis et al., 1997). Despite this finding, perceived neighborhood safety (how safe is it "for your child to play outdoors with other children in your neighborhood without adult supervision") was not predictive of change in physical activity of fourthgraders from suburban San Diego who were followed for 20 months (Sallis et al., 1999). There are many factors that affect the perception of safety outdoors, ranging from neighborhood crime levels, to traffic patterns and sidewalk availability, to playground disrepair. Research has not been conducted to determine which aspects of neighborhood safety are most relevant in the decisions made by families in WIC about spending time outdoors.

It is intuitive that parental activity would affect the activity of preschoolers, and the *Dietary Guidelines* emphasize that parents should be active with their children. Parent activity has been the most widely studied potential correlate of child physical activity, but the review of physical activity correlates by Sallis et al. (2000) did not find compelling evidence across 29 studies that parental activity and child activity were correlated. While this finding does not negate the many potential benefits of parents being active with their children, it does not support the idea that increasing a parent's activity level will necessarily increase their child's activity. Thus, there is not sufficient evidence that either the time children spend outdoors or parental physical activity levels would meet the criteria (Box 7-2) to be target behavioral indicators for physical activity in WIC-enrolled preschool children.

Television Viewing as a Behavioral Indicator of Physical Activity

Television viewing has also been considered a potential behavioral indicator of physical activity and, for several reasons, the committee felt that this indicator merited separate discussion. One reason is that the *Dietary Guidelines* address television viewing in each of the two guidelines under "Aim for Fitness": *Aim for a Healthy Weight* and *Be Physically Active Each Day*.

A second reason is the well-documented association between television viewing and obesity and the increasing problem of obesity in the populations served by WIC. Although adverse affects of television viewing on fitness and fatness may not occur until school-age or beyond, the trajectories towards television viewing habits in middle childhood appear set in children by 24 months of age and are less favorable for children whose mothers are less educated (Certain and Kahn, 2001). This makes television viewing a particular concern for the WIC population.

Several large studies, based on nationally representative samples, show a direct association between television viewing and obesity in children and adolescents (Andersen et al., 1998; Dietz and Gortmaker, 1985; Gordon-Larsen et al., 1999; Gortmaker et al., 1996; Pate and Ross, 1987). Recent experimental evidence has shown that reducing television viewing time in school-age children reduces the normal age-related increase in BMI (Robinson, 1999), suggesting that television viewing may cause obesity. As for adult women, several observational studies have also shown a direct association between television viewing and obesity (Crawford et al., 1999; Jeffery and French, 1998; Sidney et al., 1996; Tucker and Bagwell, 1991), but there have been no randomized trials that involve reducing television viewing in adults.

Despite these studies, the association between television viewing and fatness in preschoolers is less clear (DuRant et al., 1994; Klesges et al., 1995b). This could be due to the difficulty of measuring television viewing accurately in preschoolers. For example, there are no validated measures of parent-reported hours of child television viewing for preschool children, and parent reports may be subject to social desirability bias. The short attention span of young children and their proclivity for frequent but short bouts of activity may mean that many preschoolers are active while watching television (DuRant et al., 1994).

The Relationship of Television Viewing to Physical Activity and Overweight/Obesity

The interrelationships between television viewing (and other sedentary behaviors), physical activity, and obesity are complex and not yet fully understood. Despite the persistent association between television viewing and obesity, television viewing is not always highly correlated to physical activity, making it an unsuitable candidate as a behavioral indicator for physical activity. This is especially true for children (DuRant et al., 1994; Sallis et al., 2000; Strauss et al., in press) and women (Jeffery and French, 1998) in relationship to moderate or low-intensity activity.

There are at least three possible explanations for the lack of a consistent relationship between television viewing and physical activity. The most likely explanation is that the relationship between television viewing and obesity is only partly mediated by reductions in physical activity (Robinson, 1998). Television viewing has been shown to be associated with food consumption (Coon et al., 2001; Jeffery and French, 1998). Children and adults may not only be eating while watching television, but their food consumption may be influenced by the advertising (Gorn and Goldberg, 1982; Jeffrey et al., 1982; Taras and Gage, 1995). A second possibility is that television viewing substitutes for moderate or low-level activities that are difficult to measure, and television viewing is less often substituted for the vigorous activities that are more often and more accurately measured. Finally, television is just one form of sedentary activity and may not serve equally across ages, races, or cultural groups as a proxy for inactivity. Other forms of sedentary behavior in both women and preschool children, aside from television viewing, have not been well characterized.

In summary, while television viewing may be a particular form of inactivity that contributes to overweight and obesity both by reducing energy expenditure and increasing energy intake, the exact mechanism is uncertain. While television viewing may be a plausible target behavior for physical activity, more needs to be known about whether altering television viewing levels in the populations served by WIC would have a demonstrable impact on activity or fatness.

CONCLUSIONS REGARDING THE USE OF BEHAVIORAL INDICATORS FOR ELIGIBILITY DETERMINATION

Behavioral indicators of food intake or physical activity hold no promise of distinguishing individuals who are ineligible from those eligible for WIC based on the criterion *failure to meet Dietary Guidelines*, or on nutrient intake or level of physical activity. However, assessment methods and behavioral indicators do offer promise of improving the understanding of diet and activity behaviors of WIC participants as a group, which could be used to design effective nutrition education programs that target behavior change related to the *Dietary Guidelines*. Likewise, behavioral indicators hold promise for monitoring the dietary intake and physical activity levels of groups and thereby evaluation of program effectiveness. Research efforts should focus on determining the feasibility and validity of assessing target behavioral indicators for diet and physical activity in the population served by WIC.

8

Evidence of Dietary Risk Among Low-Income Women and Children

The preceding chapters have discussed the poor reliability and validity of methods used to assess the diet and physical activity in *individuals*. This chapter addresses the nutritional vulnerability of pregnant and postpartum women and children as *groups* and presents results from relevant dietary intake studies as well as relationships between income and dietary risk. A discussion of infants has been omitted since this report does not cover dietary risk for this high-risk group.

NUTRITIONAL VULNERABILITY OF GROUPS SERVED BY WIC

Pregnant and Lactating Women

The need for food energy and the Estimated Average Requirements (EARs) for most nutrients are higher for pregnant and lactating women than they are for other women in the childbearing years (IOM, 2001). At the same time, the effects of nutrient shortfalls potentially are more serious for pregnant and lactating women than for other women. Both the woman's health and that of the embryo, developing fetus, or infant may be affected. For example, inadequate energy intake may contribute to low gestational weight gain and fetal growth restriction. Likewise, inadequate iron intake may lead to maternal anemia and to low iron stores in the infant. The combination of higher requirements and/or higher recommended nutrient densities and more serious results of deficiency means that pregnant and lactating women are more vulnerable to nutrition problems than are other adults—both women and men. For example, iron deficiency is nearly twice as prevalent among low-income women in their reproductive years, in comparison with those who are more advantaged (Looker et al., 1997), but the three tests required to determine iron deficiency are not a routine part of health care or of WIC services.

In addition, mounting evidence indicates that practices during pregnancy may have a long-term impact on health. For example, periconceptional intake of folic acid is important not only in the prevention of central nervous system and other birth defects but also in reducing the risk of cancer and other chronic disease in later life (Toren et al., 1996). Likewise, increasing maternal intake of omega-3 fatty acids is associated with increased gestation duration (Allen and Harris, 2001), improved fetal neurological development (Innis, 2000), and lowered maternal cardiovascular risk (Mori and Beilin, 2001).

Postpartum, Nonlactating Women

Little attention has been paid to maternal nutrition after pregnancy, particularly among women who are not lactating, possibly because they have had a low priority for receipt of WIC services. Two studies were identified that address postpartum, nonlactating women. Caan and colleagues (1987) examined the influence of extended maternal food supplementation (5–7 months) in the interpregnancy interval compared with more limited supplementation (0–2 months). All women received WIC benefits during both the index and subsequent pregnancies. In comparison to those with limited feeding, women with extended supplementation had significantly improved outcomes in the subsequent pregnancy: birth length was increased by 0.3 cm and birth weight was 120 g higher after controlling for gestational duration and other potential confounding variables (e.g., maternal smoking and the birth weight of the prior infant). Maternal iron status was improved—hemoglobin levels were increased significantly, on average by 0.3 mg/dL with extended feeding. In addition, risk of maternal overweight and obesity (defined as > 120 percent of ideal weight in this study) was reduced twofold among women on extended supplementation (Caan et al., 1987). Pehrsson and coworkers (2001) examined three indicators of iron status among postpartum, nonlactating participants and eligible nonparticipants (women unserved because of lack of funds). Women who participated in WIC for the full 6 months were significantly less likely to become anemic than were the eligible nonparticipants.

Young Children

The years prior to age 5 are a time of rapid growth and development. The results of a shortfall during the first 4 years of life can be very serious, including both stunted physical growth and cognitive deficits. Compared with children from more affluent families, low-income children are more likely to have anemia (CDC, 1998a), to be stunted and/or overweight (CDC, 1998a), to have higher blood lead levels (NCHS, 1998) and, perhaps in consequence, to be developmentally delayed or learning disabled (Brooks-Gunne and Duncan, 1997). They also are more likely to have experienced hunger in the past year and to come from a family where the head of household reports fear of going out into the neighborhood (Brooks-Gunne and Duncan, 1997).

Risk of Becoming Overweight or Obese

Prevalence of Overweight and Obesity

Over the past few decades, overweight and obesity have become more prevalent among women in the childbearing years (Flegal et al., 1998; Kuczmarski et al., 1994; Mokdad et al., 1999) and among young children in the population as a whole (Ogden et al., 1997). Overweight and obesity are more prevalent in lower- than in higher-income groups (NCHS, 1998), as well as in the subgroups of the population that give rise to many of those who are eligible for WIC (Must et al., 1999). Thus, it is reasonable to expect that the prevalence of overweight and obesity would be higher in populations served by WIC. In 1990, 19 percent of pregnant women in WIC were obese (Kim et al., 1992)[1]; but by 1994, the prevalence of obesity had increased to 22 percent (Randall et al., 1995). A more recent analysis of data on pregnant women enrolled in the Ohio and Kentucky WIC programs, using current adult criteria for obesity (BMI $\geq$ 30 kg/m^2) and overweight (BMI $\geq$ 25 kg/m^2) (NIH, 1998; WHO, 1995), showed that during the first trimester of pregnancy, over one-fourth of all women and one-third of African-American women were obese (Whitaker et al., 1997, 2001). Few data are available on the extent to which those who enter pregnancy at a healthy weight become overweight during pregnancy or the postpartum period. However, excessive weight gain during pregnancy may be a factor that increases the risk of new postpartum overweight and obesity among young and mature gravidas in general (Gunderson et al., 2000; Scholl et al., 1996).

Among 4-year-old children in WIC, the prevalence of overweight (weight-for-height $\geq$ ninety-fifth percentile) increased from 8.2 percent in 1983 to 10.6 percent in 1995, a relative increase of almost one-third in just 12 years (Mei et al., 1998). Other recent analyses of data on children enrolled in the Ohio and Kentucky WIC programs (Whitaker, personal communication) in 1998 have used the 2000 Centers for Disease Control and Prevention growth charts

---

[1] Defined at that time as a prepregnant BMI of $\geq$ 29 kg/m^2 in accordance with the cut points recommended by a prior committee (IOM, 1990).

(Kuczmarski et al., 2000) to estimate the proportion of 4-year-olds at risk for overweight (BMI ≥ eighty-fifth and < ninety-fifth percentile) and overweight (BMI ≥ ninety-fifth percentile). Across these two states, the prevalence of at risk for overweight and overweight among children 48 to 60 months of age were 14 percent and 12 percent, respectively. Although this could be interpreted as saying that WIC is making things worse, there is no reason to believe that this increased prevalence of overweight is isolated to those enrolled in WIC or is somehow caused by WIC. Examination of nationally representative cross-sectional surveys of 4- and 5-year-olds in the United States has shown that the rate of overweight (weight-for-height ≥ ninety-fifth percentile) nearly doubled from 5.8 to 10 percent between 1971 and 1994 (Ogden et al., 1997). Similar increases are also being seen among preschool children in other developed countries (Bundred et al., 2001).

Relationship of Income and Food Security to the Risk of Overweight or Obesity

Because the problem of obesity disproportionately affects low-income women and because the prevalence of obesity has increased substantially in low-income children in recent years, it might appear that food supplementation in WIC is a counterproductive strategy for preventing or treating the problem of obesity in WIC. However, there is no evidence that enrollment in the WIC Program is a risk factor for obesity among income-eligible children. In fact, low-income children enrolled in WIC do not appear to have higher weight-for-height than those low-income children not enrolled in WIC (CDC, 1996).

There is also a poorly understood paradox that food insecurity and obesity can coexist. Food insecure women are more likely to be overweight than those who are food secure (Olson, 1999; Townsend et al., 2001), and this appears to be true even within the population of women receiving food stamps (Townsend et al., 2001). The question of whether children living in more food-insecure households are more likely to be overweight has not yet been addressed using the current U.S. Department of Agriculture Food Security Scale (Gleason et al., 2000). However, Alaimo and colleagues, in a series of analyses using data from the Third National Health and Nutrition Examination Survey, have examined several child outcomes in relation to household food insufficiency (living in a family that reports "sometimes or often not getting enough food to eat")—a state thought to be different and more adverse than food insecurity (Carleson and Briefel, 1995). Although there was no tendency for household food insufficiency to increase the risk of overweight in 2- to 7-year-old children (Alaimo et al., 2001b), school-age children living in food-insufficient households have been shown to have poorer parent-reported health status (Alaimo et al., 2001c) and poorer outcomes on certain measures of cognitive, academic, and psychosocial development, after controlling for other socioeconomic indicators (Alaimo et al., 2001a).

Thus, the above current evidence suggests that food supplementation may decrease, rather than increase, the risk of overweight among food-insecure mothers in WIC and that it may promote varied aspects of health and well-being among food-insufficient children without adding to the risk of overweight.

Health Risks of Overweight and Obesity in Mothers and Children

Maternal overweight and obesity are associated with a reduced risk of fetal growth restriction but have serious consequences for maternal health and other aspects of fetal well-being. Risks of maternal hypertension, gestational diabetes, and cesarean section increase with increasing BMI; hospitalization expenses increase as well (Galtier-Dereure et al., 1995). Risk of late fetal death is increased twofold in women who are obese before pregnancy (BMI $\geq$ 30). In nulliparas, fetal death is increased threefold in the overweight and fivefold in the obese and there are trends suggesting a rise in both early neonatal death and very preterm delivery ($<$ 32 weeks) with increasing maternal pregravid BMI (Cnattingus et al, 1998). A similar effect on mortality was observed as part of the Collaborative Perinatal Project: perinatal mortality was increased approximately twofold among overweight gravidas (BMI 25–30) and more than threefold among those who were obese (BMI $>$ 30) (Naeye, 1990). Maternal pregravid obesity also is a risk factor for major congenital defects in the fetus (Naeye, 1990). The well-known protective effect of folic acid intake on risk of neural tube defects appears to be absent among obese women (Shaw et al., 1996; Waller et al., 1994; Werler et al., 1996). While the reasons for this effect have yet to be identified, a similar lack of benefit was observed with zinc and obesity: risk of low birth weight was decreased in normal weight, but not in obese women receiving supplemental zinc (Goldenberg et al., 1995).

Overweight children are more likely to become obese adults (Power, 1997; Serdula et al., 1993). By 6 to 9 years of age, an overweight child with an obese parent has more than a 70 percent chance of being obese in young adulthood (Whitaker et al., 1997). At any age, once obesity develops, it is very difficult to treat (Barlow and Dietz, 1998; NIH Technology Assessment Conference Panel, 1993). Even in childhood, being overweight is associated with abnormalities in cardiovascular disease risk factors such as blood pressure, serum lipid concentrations, and serum insulin concentrations (Freedman et al., 1999). There are now alarming increases in the prevalence of Type II diabetes among young adults (Mokdad et al., 2000) and adolescents (Fagot-Campagna et al., 2000) that are attributable to the problem of obesity early in life. For all these reasons, there is great interest in preventing children from ever becoming overweight.

Implications for WIC

Because WIC serves almost 6 million children under 5 years of age, the program has a unique opportunity to provide the early intervention required to prevent childhood obesity. Anthropometric measurements in WIC identify applicants at nutritional risk because of overweight or obesity. While there are no highly accurate methods to determine which normal weight infants and children in WIC are likely to become overweight, it is clear that both maternal and sibling obesity substantially (and independently) increase the risk that a newborn in WIC will become overweight by 4 years of age (Whitaker et al., 2001). This population of newborns may be a promising target group for developing obesity prevention strategies in WIC. However, these strategies will require a new nutrition counseling paradigm that takes into account the evidence that many families in WIC with already overweight children may not believe that their children are overweight (Baughcum et al., 2000; Jain et al., 2001). Furthermore, the paradigm will need to consider the important role of activity, along with diet, in obesity prevention.

RESULTS FROM RELEVANT DIETARY INTAKE STUDIES

No representative studies have reported on the nutrients or foods consumed by the women and children applying for WIC. Thus, indirect data must be used to examine the potential dietary risk of these groups. Relatively little information is available about dietary intake of pregnant or lactating women or postpartum women for the 6-month period after delivery, which makes the data even more indirect for these groups. This section covers dietary intake information about women and children in general, and about those served by WIC.

Dietary Intake of the General Population

Intakes Below the Estimated Average Requirement

For most nutrients, the recommended method to assess the adequacy of nutrient intake by a population is a three-step process:

1. Obtain estimates of the usual intake distribution of the population. This requires at least two nonconsecutive days of research-quality diet recalls or records from a representative sample of the population of interest.
2. Make statistical adjustments of the data to remove within person variation in intake.
3. Determine the percentage of the population with usual intakes above or below the Estimated Average Requirement (EAR) (IOM, 2000a).

For iron, because the distribution of requirements is skewed, the probability approach should be used as described by the Institute of Medicine (IOM, 2000a, 2001; NRC, 1986).

No studies were found reporting percentages of individuals with intakes below the EAR for age or physiological status. Therefore, to identify problem nutrients, the committee used tables of percentiles for usual intakes of nutrients from food published in IOM reports on Dietary Reference Intakes (IOM, 1997, 1998, 2000b, 2001) and the EARs for young children and women by physiologic status. The dietary intake data used for those tables are from the 1994–1996 Continuing Survey of Food Intakes by Individuals (CSFII) for phosphorus and magnesium and from the 1988–1994 Third National Health and Nutrition Examination Survey (NHANES III) for the remaining nutrients. This method allowed the identification of a range for the percentage of individuals with intakes below the EAR. Three nutrients were excluded: calcium, for which an EAR has not been set; folate, for which current intakes are likely to be higher than reported because of the fortification of enriched cereal grains and the use of micrograms of dietary folate equivalents for setting the EAR (IOM, 1998); and iron, for which appropriate data are lacking.

Nutrients for which more than 5 percent of the age group has an intake less than the EAR are shown in Table 8-1. No data are available to determine the extent to which persons who are categorically and income-eligible for WIC are represented in the group with intakes below the EAR, but data covered in a later section, "Associations of Food Intake with Income," suggest that they may be at increased risk.

Estimation of the Percentage of WIC Applicants at Dietary Risk

In a report to the U.S. Department of Agriculture that addressed the estimation of dietary risk (and other components of nutritional risk), Sigma One Corporation (2000) used 1-day dietary intake data from Phase 1 of NHANES III (1988–1991) for women ages 17 to 49 years and children ages 1 to 4 years. The cut points shown in Table 8-2 represent modal levels used to determine dietary adequacy obtained from 1997 WIC state plans. The cut points are similar to, but not coincident with, the recommended number of servings for each food group specified by the Food Guide Pyramid. Since only approximately 6 percent of the women studied had intakes that met or exceeded the cut point for each food group, Sigma One concluded that 94 percent of the women were at dietary risk. Reported intakes by children ages 1 to 4 years were somewhat better: 15 percent met modal intake for each food group placing 85 percent at dietary risk.

TABLE 8-1 Nutrients for Which More than 5 Percent of the Age Group has an Intake less than the Estimated Average Requirement (EAR)

Nutrient	Age Group (yr)	Percentile with Intake Below the EAR
Phosphorus	14–18	25–50
Magnesium	14–30	75–90
	31–50	50–75
	Pregnant, all ages	50
Zinc	14–18	25
	29–50	25–50
	Pregnant, all ages	25–50
Vitamin A	1–3	10–25
	14–18	10–25
	19–50	25–50
	Pregnant, all ages	> 25
Vitamin C	14–50	10–25
Vitamin B_6	14–18	15–25
	19–50	10–15
	Pregnant, all ages	25–50

NOTE: Estimates for lactating women could not be determined with the available data.
SOURCE: IOM (1997, 1998, 2000b, 2001)

TABLE 8-2 Cutoff Values Used by Sigma One Corporation to Identify Dietary Risk, by Participant Category and Food Group

	Number of Servings by Participant Category				
Food Category	Pregnant Women	Lactating Women	Postpartum Women	Children Ages 1–3 yr[a]	Children Age 4 yr[a]
Milk products	3	3	2	4	4
Meat and beans group	3	3	2	2	2
Grains	6	6	6	6	6
Total fruits and vegetables	5	5	5	5	5
Vitamin A foods	1	1	1	1	1
Vitamin C foods	1	1	1	1	1
Other fruits and vegetables	3	3	3	3	3

[a] Serving size typically equals one-half of the adult serving, except for the milk group.
SOURCE: Sigma One Corporation (2000).

Percentages Meeting Food Serving Recommendations of the Food Guide Pyramid

Krebs-Smith and colleagues (1997) conducted a similar but more rigorous analysis of the food group intake of adults. They determined the percentages who met energy and age-based Food Guide Pyramid recommendations (see Table 3-2) using 3 days of dietary data from the 1989–1991 CSFII. Only 0.1 percent of the women met the recommendations for all five basic food groups. Notably, the average age of the men and women who met all the recommendations was 60 years—well beyond the childbearing years. In another study of women ages 18 to 39 years, nearly 34 percent had fewer than 2.5 servings of fruits and vegetables per day (LSRO/FASEB, 1995). Munoz and coworkers (1997), in a rigorous analysis of 1989–1991 CSFII data, found that none of the children ages 2 to 5 years ($n = 1,028$) met the minimum recommendations for all five food groups, after allowing for smaller portion sizes of grains, fruits, vegetables, and meats. Considering the five food groups individually, recommendations for the meat group were least likely to be met—only about 13 percent of the children met them. A much smaller ($n = 110$) but similar study of older children (ages 7 to 14 years) conducted in Alabama found that only 5 percent and 9 percent met Pyramid recommendations for fruit and milk products, respectively, over 3 days. Moreover, the mean proportion of calories from fat was well above the recommended 30 percent for children ages 2 to 5 years (CDC, 1996), suggesting that a high percentage of preschool children do not meet the recommendation. Based on data from NHANES III (1988–1994), only about 23 percent of children ages 2 to 5 years met the dietary recommendation for total fat intake (Troiano et al., 2000).

Studies Using the Healthy Eating Index

Bowman and colleagues compared the Healthy Eating Index (HEI; see Chapter 5) of selected groups using 2 days of 1994–1996 CSFII data from subjects of all ages. (A score of 80 or more implies a good diet.) African Americans had lower HEI scores than other ethnic groups (59 compared with 64–67). Children ages 2 to 3 years had a higher mean HEI score (74) than did older children (68 for children ages 4 to 6 years) or women in the childbearing years (61–62). McCullough et al. (2000) used data from Food Frequency Questionnaires obtained in the Nurses' Health Study to calculate HEI scores and found that only 1 to 2 percent of the 67,272 subjects (many of whom are beyond the childbearing years) had an HEI score greater than 90.

Dietary Intake of Groups Served by WIC

Women and children participating in WIC have intakes of energy and certain nutrients that exceed those of nonparticipants (Rush, 1988; Suitor et al., 1990). While data are lacking to determine whether the changes resulted from WIC participation, it is reasonable to infer that intakes while served by WIC are at least as high and probably higher than intakes of new applicants. Participants have consistently reported food intakes that resulted in protein intakes at or above the 1989 Recommended Dietary Allowances (Kramer-LeBlanc et al., 1999). Data from this study are not available on the percentages of participants whose intakes were below the EARs for nutrients. However, nutrients identified as problematic included calcium, iron, folic acid, zinc, and magnesium during pregnancy; vitamin C and zinc during lactation; and iron, calcium, and magnesium in nonbreastfeeding, postpartum women. The overall diet of pregnant and postpartum WIC participants tended to be low in calories (a mean of 70–89 percent of the recommended energy allowance) with a low nutrient density and 33–37 percent of calories from fat—well above the recommended 30 percent. Mean intakes for the WIC target nutrients were fairly similar for WIC participants, income-eligible nonparticipants, and the total sample of pregnant, lactating, and postpartum women (Kramer-LeBlanc et al., 1999). In some instances (e.g., folic acid, B_6), however, their intakes were higher than those of the comparison groups of income-eligible individuals not participating in WIC or of the total sample in the same age range.

Dietary data from 332 pregnant women participating in the 1988–1994 NHANES III (Mardis and Anand, 2000) were examined for WIC participants, for income-eligible nonparticipants, and for those whose incomes exceed the threshold for WIC. On average, all groups consumed less than the recommended number of servings from the Food Guide Pyramid based upon a 2,200 kcal diet as shown in Table 3-2 (using three servings as the cut-off value from the milk group). However, each group consumed more than the recommended percentage of energy from fat and saturated fat and more than 2,400 mg of sodium. In addition, WIC participants consumed significantly fewer servings of milk than did the women with incomes greater than 185 percent of poverty.

ASSOCIATIONS OF FOOD INTAKE WITH INCOME

Dietary data show an inverse relationship between income and dietary intake of energy and of certain food groups. For example, children from low-income households (< 131 percent of poverty) are less likely to meet current recommendations for the consumption of fruit and milk products than are those from more affluent families (Munoz et al., 1997). Likewise, lower-income adults (women and minorities in particular) are over-represented among the group whose diets fail to meet any of the recommendations for food consumption in the Food Guide Pyramid (Krebs-Smith et al., 1997). The percentage of women who report the consumption of fruit during 3 days increases with increasing income level (LSRO/FASEB, 1995).

On average, children in poverty have higher fat intakes than those in more affluent families (USDA, 1999). Smaller percentages of low-income (< 131 percent of poverty) children ages 3 to 5 years met recommendations for total fat than did those whose household incomes were 131 to 350 percent and over 350 percent of poverty (21 percent, 34 percent, and 44 percent, respectively). Similarly, only about 12 percent of the lowest-income children met recommendations for saturated fat intake compared with about 25 percent of the children at 131 to 350 percent of poverty and about 31 percent of the higher-income children.

Block and Abrams (1993) used data from the second NHANES and from the CSFII to examine associations of nutrient and food intakes with income. They found that women with incomes near poverty or below poverty had lower mean intakes for every nutrient examined (protein, calcium, folic acid, iron, zinc, vitamins A, C , E, and B_6). Low-income women, in particular, ate few fruits and vegetables. About half ate no vegetables at all, including potatoes, when surveyed over four nonsuccessive days. In a random sample of mothers in a rural New York county, nearly 75 percent of the food-insecure mothers (n = 103) reported 0 to 2 servings of fruits and vegetables daily, compared with 55 percent of the food-secure mothers (n = 90) (Kendall et al., 1996).

Scores from summary measures such as the HEI improve with increased income, in part because of increased variety of intake with increased income. Based on 1994–1996 CSFII data for all ages, people with household incomes at or below 50 percent of poverty had average variety scores of 6.9 (out of a possible 10), whereas those with household incomes at or above 300 percent of poverty had average variety scores of 7.9. Those from the lowest-income households also had lower average scores for saturated fat (5.7) and sodium (6.6) than did people whose household income was more than three times the poverty level (saturated fat, 6.6; sodium, 7.9) (Bowman et al., 1998).

Findings from the Dietary Quality Index, an overall score determined by whether or not an individual's diet met recommendations for fat (total, saturated), cholesterol, fruits and vegetables, complex carbohydrate, protein, sodium, and calcium (NRC, 1989) were similar—higher income was associated with better scores. Those whose diets were judged as "poor" had lower incomes and were 5 to 7 times more likely not to be college graduates than those with diets classified as "good" (Patterson et al., 1994).

Throughout history, it has been observed that people restrict their food selection as food prices rise (Karp and Greene, 1983). In the instance of the United States oil embargo that occurred in the 1970s, the prevalence of anemia increased among poor urban children when a major source of iron (meat) began to disappear from the family diet due to the rising cost of food (Karp and Greene, 1983). Thus, when income falls and food selection is sufficiently narrow, dietary quality suffers and nutritional status frequently will worsen, particularly among the poor.

SUMMARY OF EVIDENCE SUGGESTING DIETARY RISK

Box 8-1 summarizes the broad range of evidence suggesting that individuals who are both categorically and income-eligible for WIC participation generally are also at dietary risk. The need for energy and for most nutrients is increased during pregnancy and lactation; thus, the effects of low intake are more serious for pregnant and lactating women than for other women.

When there is a shortfall, the health of both mother and fetus is likely to be affected. Likewise, the years prior to age 5 are a time of rapid growth and development. The results of a shortfall during the first 4 years of life can be very serious, including stunted physical growth and cognitive deficits. The inverse relationship between quality of intake and income is well documented. The diets of many low-income women and children are of a low nutrient density, contain more fat and saturated fat than recommended by the *Dietary Guidelines*, and fail to meet food group recommendations specified by the Food Guide Pyramid, especially in the fruit and vegetable groups. These data suggest that essentially all women and children who are income-eligible for WIC are at dietary risk.

BOX 8-1 Summary of Evidence Suggesting Dietary Risk for Categorically and Income-Eligible WIC Applicants[a]

- Less than 1 percent of all women meet recommendations for all five Pyramid groups (Krebs-Smith et al., 1997).
- Less than 1 percent of children ages 2 to 5 years meet recommendations for all five Pyramid groups (Munoz et al., 1997).
- The percentage of women consuming fruit during 3 days of intake increases with increasing income level (LSRO/FASEB, 1995).
- Members of low-income households are less likely to meet recommendations for fruit (adults and children) and for milk products (children) than are more affluent households (Mardis and Anand, 2000).
- Food-insecure mothers are less likely to meet recommendations for fruit and vegetable intake than are food-secure mothers (Kendall et al., 1996).
- The percentage of children meeting recommendations for fat and saturated fat as a percentage of food energy increases with increasing income level (USDA, 1999).
- Low-income individuals and African Americans have lower mean Healthy Eating Index scores than do other income and racial/ethnic groups (Bowman et al., 1998).

[a] While representative data with regard to pregnant and postpartum women is lacking, their risk is likely to be higher than that of nonpregnant, nonlactating women.

9

Findings and Recommendations

Methods to identify and determine eligibility based on dietary risk of applicants have presented a challenge to WIC for many years. This report builds on the recommendation of the report, *WIC Nutrition Risk Criteria* (IOM, 1996), which recommended using *failure to meet Dietary Guidelines* as a risk criterion for WIC eligibility and also recommended research to develop practical and valid assessment tools. The current committee evaluated available dietary assessment methods, scientific literature regarding the tools these methods employ, and the strengths and limitations of these methods and tools to establish eligibility for WIC based on dietary risk. This chapter provides a summary of the committee's major findings and a recommendation regarding the determination of eligibility for WIC based on two types of dietary risk: *failure to meet Dietary Guidelines* and *inadequate diet*. The chapter also identifies appropriate uses for assessment data on both dietary intake and physical activity within the WIC program.

FINDINGS

Basing Risk Criteria on the *Dietary Guidelines* for Americans

Focusing on the single guideline *Let The Pyramid Guide Your Food Choices* was determined to be the most feasible, comprehensive, and objective approach to using the *Dietary Guidelines* for establishing dietary risk for those individuals 2 years of age and older. A majority of state WIC agencies already use some version of this approach as the basis for setting a criterion that addresses the dietary risk *failure to meet Dietary Guidelines*. Based on review of the *Dietary Guidelines* (USDA/HHS, 2000) and the scientific underpinnings of the Food Guide Pyramid (USDA, 1992), the committee determined that this approach should use the recommended number of servings based on energy needs as the cut-off point for each of the five basic food groups (see Table 3-2). For example, the criterion for active, pregnant, adult women would be at least nine servings from the grains group.

> **Finding 1.** A dietary risk criterion that uses the WIC applicant's usual intake of the five basic Pyramid food groups as the indicator and the recommended numbers of servings based on energy needs as the cut-off points is consistent with *failure to meet Dietary Guidelines*.

Prevalence of Dietary Risk Based on the Food Guide Pyramid Recommendations

In the United States, more than 96 percent of individuals, and an even higher percentage of low-income individuals (such as those served by WIC), do not usually consume the recommended number of servings specified by the Food Guide Pyramid (Krebs-Smith et al., 1997; Munoz et al., 1997). Thus, the identification of individuals who are *not* at dietary risk becomes highly problematic.

> Finding 2. Nearly all U.S. women and children usually consume fewer than the recommended number of servings specified by the Food Guide Pyramid and, therefore, would be at dietary risk based on the criterion *failure to meet Dietary Guidelines* that is described in Finding 1.

Food-Based Assessment of Dietary Intake

Nutritional status and health are influenced by usual or long-term dietary intake. For this reason, dietary assessment for establishing WIC eligibility should be based on usual intake. Day-to-day variation in food and nutrient intake by individuals is so large in the United States that one or two 24-hour diet recalls or food records cannot provide accurate information about an individual's usual intake. In the WIC setting, it is impractical to obtain more than one or two recalls or records under standardized conditions that would promote accurate reporting. Moreover, most people make many errors when reporting their food intake because of the complex nature of the task. These errors increase the likelihood that eligibility status for WIC will be misclassified in the category of dietary risk.

Food frequency questionnaires (FFQs) are designed to assess usual intake and may be practical to administer to many WIC clients. However, they are subject to many types of errors, and their performance characteristics are unsatisfactory for determining individual eligibility. For example, when reported food or nutrient intakes from an FFQ are compared with the values obtained using a large number of research-quality diet recalls or food records, correlations generally range between 0.3 and 0.7. Although correlations in that range may be considered satisfactory for making inferences about intakes by groups of individuals in epidemiologic research, such data cannot accurately classify individuals as above or below set cut-off points—a serious problem when the goal is determining the eligibility of an individual. Shortening FFQs generally makes them more responsive to operational constraints, but further reduces their accuracy and utility.

Few practical methods have been developed or tested that compare food intakes with the *Dietary Guidelines* or Food Guide Pyramid recommendations. Such methods would require converting amounts of each type of food consumed to Pyramid portions to determine whether the Pyramid recommendations had been met. This is a complex process, especially for mixed dishes, and does not lend itself to operational constraints in the WIC setting.

> **Finding 3.** Even research-quality dietary assessment methods are not sufficiently accurate or precise to distinguish an individual's eligibility status using criteria based on the Food Guide Pyramid or on nutrient intake.

Physical Activity Assessment

The committee considered physical activity assessment as a part of dietary risk assessment for two reasons. First, the *Dietary Guidelines* include a quantitative recommendation for physical activity levels for adults and for children 2 years of age and older. Second, WIC has a mandate to focus on primary prevention, including the primary prevention of overweight and obesity. Overweight and obesity are now major health concerns among those served by WIC, and proper risk assessment for prevention or treatment must consider both diet and physical activity.

Physical activity assessment relates to two of the *Dietary Guidelines* (*Aim For A Healthy Weight* and *Be Physically Active Each Day*) and thus could potentially be used as another way to define *failure to meet Dietary Guidelines*. The physical activity guideline specifies "Aim to accumulate at least 30 minutes (adults) or 60 minutes (children) of moderate physical activity most days of the week, preferably daily." These specifications could be used as WIC eligibility criteria under the dietary risk subgroup *failure to meet Dietary Guidelines.*

A review of the literature found no physical activity assessment instruments that meet the operational constraints of WIC and that also can accurately and reliably assess whether a woman or child is obtaining at least the specified amount of physical activity. Because of the inherent cognitive challenge of accurately recalling and characterizing the varied activity behaviors that together constitute an individual's physical activity level, it is unlikely that there could ever be a practical instrument to establish WIC eligibility accurately based on the physical activity recommendation in the *Dietary Guidelines*.

> **Finding 4.** Physical activity assessment methods are not sufficiently accurate or reliable to distinguish individuals who are ineligible from those who are eligible for WIC services based on the physical activity component of the *Dietary Guidelines*.

Behavioral Indicators of Diet and Physical Activity

Because certain behaviors are correlated with dietary intake and physical activity, interest has arisen in the use of behavior-based assessment as a method of identifying those who usually fail to meet the *Dietary Guidelines*. Such assessment would require the identification of behavioral indicators that could distinguish individuals who meet the *Dietary Guidelines* from those who do not. The committee considered two types of behavioral indicators: surrogate and target. Surrogate behaviors are behaviors that are correlated with one or more aspects of diet or physical activity and could be used to make inferences about what children eat or how much activity they engage in. For example, the frequency of eating meals together as a family could indicate the adequacy of vegetable consumption. Target behaviors are behaviors that make good targets for change. Making changes in a target behavior would be expected to result in changes in dietary intake. Target behavioral indicators are not suitable for eligibility determination unless they also are surrogate indicators. Building on the example above, if families could be encouraged to eat meals together more frequently, and if family meals resulted in improved dietary intake, then frequency of eating meals as a family would be both a surrogate indicator and a potential target indicator for change. By analogy, if families could spend more time outdoors and if this change resulted in increased levels of physical activity, then time spent outdoors could be both a surrogate and target indicator for physical activity.

A review of the literature found few studies of behavioral correlates of diet or physical activity conducted among the groups served by WIC. No strong evidence was found that any examined behaviors would be both adequately reliable and accurate as surrogate or target behavioral indicators.

> **Finding 5.** Behavioral indicators have weak relationships with dietary or physical activity outcomes of interest. As a result, they hold no promise of distinguishing individuals who are ineligible for WIC from those who are eligible in the category of dietary risk.

RECOMMENDATION

Based on the above findings, the following recommendation is made:

Presume that all women and children ages 2 to 5 years who meet the eligibility requirements of income, categorical, and residency status also meet the requirement of nutrition risk through the category of dietary risk based on *failure to meet Dietary Guidelines*, where *failure to meet Dietary Guidelines* is defined as consuming fewer than the recommended number of servings from one or more of the five basic food groups (grains, fruits, vegetables, milk products, and meat or beans) based on an individual's estimated energy needs.

Studies suggest that nearly all women in the childbearing years and children ages 2 years and older are at dietary risk because they fail to meet the *Dietary Guidelines* as translated by recommendations of the Food Guide Pyramid (Krebs-Smith et al., 1997; Munoz et al., 1997). (See Table 3-2 for the recommended number of servings based on an individual's energy needs.) Tools currently used for dietary risk assessment appear to have very high sensitivity in that they identify nearly everyone as failing to meet the *Dietary Guidelines*, but low specificity—poor ability to identify persons who are not at dietary risk. No known dietary or physical activity assessment methods or behavioral indicators of diet or physical activity hold promise of accurately identifying the small percentage of women and children who do meet the proposed criterion based on the Food Guide Pyramid or the physical activity recommendation. Even if the percentage of individuals who meet the criterion were to increase substantially, it remains unlikely that methods can be found or developed to differentiate risk among individuals.

When WIC was originally established in 1972, the categorical groups that WIC serves were selected because of their vulnerability to nutritional insults and WIC's potential for preventing nutrition-related problems. Nutritional status and dietary intake have both short- and long-term effects on the health of the woman and on the growth, development, and health of the fetus, infant, or child. The groups served by WIC also are at increased risk of morbidity and mortality from virtually every disorder listed among the leading causes of death in the United States (cardiovascular disease, cancer, diabetes, and digestive diseases). The high prevalence of overweight and obesity and of diets that are inconsistent with the *Dietary Guidelines* (e.g., low intakes of fruits and vegetables, high intakes of saturated fats) may contribute to these increased risks.

This recommendation is not intended to affect the current use of other nutritional risk criteria for eligibility determination. That is, information should continue to be collected for the identification of other nutrition risks (e.g., hemoglobin or hematocrit to identify risk of anemia, height and weight to identify anthropometric risk, and the presence of diabetes mellitus to identify medical risk). Such information is useful for nutrition education, and it is essential to implement the priority system. As discussed in Chapter 1, when funds are insufficient to enroll all those eligible for WIC, the priority system is used to determine those at greatest need. If dietary information is collected in the WIC setting for food package tailoring, nutrition education, and/or health referrals, the methods used should be approached with caution given the likelihood of error and misclassification.

Optimal Collection and Use of Dietary and Physical Activity Data

Although individual-level reporting errors greatly reduce the validity of data for assessing diet or physical activity levels in individuals, the errors are less serious in group assessments. Moreover, a variety of statistical procedures can adjust for known sources of error (IOM, 2000a; Traub, 1994) and thereby provide reasonable tests of relationships. Thus, while identified relationships may not be true for any specific individual, they would be true for the group. For example, FFQs and recalls can be used to identify dietary patterns in a WIC population and patterns needing improvement. Repeated collection of dietary recalls or FFQs also may be used to monitor change over time at the group level or to assess effects of nutrition education interventions.

Findings from such analyses could be used to design nutrition education programs and monitor their effectiveness. For example, diet recalls can provide valid information on the average intakes of groups, assuming that a standardized data collection approach is used and an adequate sample size (50 or larger) is available. If more than one recall is collected on at least a subsample of the group and appropriate adjustments are made, one could determine the proportion of the group with usual nutrient intakes that are less than the Estimated Average Requirement (IOM, 2000a). Group dietary intake information for a WIC population (e.g., data from a recent national dietary survey such as the National Health and Nutrition Examination Survey or the Continuing Survey of Food

Intake by Individuals or data collected in a special WIC study) could be used to identify areas for targeted nutrition education services.

Likewise, physical activity assessment tools may be sufficiently valid to assess physical activity levels within groups. These data would be valuable for monitoring groups of individuals or target populations within WIC that may be at higher risk for low physical activity levels and that may benefit most from interventions within WIC to increase physical activity levels.

Group assessment data would best be collected by trained individuals on randomly selected subsamples of the WIC population. However, any tool used for this purpose still must be evaluated in terms of the criteria presented in Chapter 4 (e.g., a tool would still need to be easy to administer, appropriate for the group, and reasonably accurate).

CONCLUDING REMARK

In summary, evidence exists to conclude that nearly all low-income women in the childbearing years and children ages 2 to 5 years are at dietary risk, are vulnerable to nutrition insults, and may benefit from WIC's services. Further, due to the complex nature of dietary patterns, it is unlikely that a tool will be developed to fulfill its intended purpose within WIC: to classify individuals accurately with respect to their true dietary risk. Thus, any tools adopted would result in misclassification of the eligibility status of some, potentially many, individuals. By presuming that all who meet the categorical and income eligibility requirements are at dietary risk, WIC retains its potential for preventing and correcting nutrition-related problems while avoiding serious misclassification errors that could lead to denial of services to eligible individuals.

10

References

Ainsworth BE. 2000a. Challenges in measuring physical activity in women. *Exerc Sport Sci Rev* 28:93–96.
Ainsworth BE. 2000b. Issues in the assessment of physical activity in women. *Res Q Exerc Sport* 71:S37–S42.
Ainsworth BE, Jacobs DR Jr, Leon AS. 1993a. Validity and reliability of self-reported physical activity status: The Lipid Research Clinics questionnaire. *Med Sci Sports Exerc* 25:92–98.
Ainsworth BE, Richardson M, Jacobs DR, Leon AS. 1993b. Gender differences in physical activity. *Women Sport Phys Activ J* 2:1–16.
Ainsworth BE, Irwin ML, Addy CL, Whitt MC, Stolarczyk LM. 1999. Moderate physical activity patterns of minority women: The Cross-Cultural Activity Participation Study. *J Womens Health Gend Based Med* 8:805–813.
Ajani UA, Willett WC, Seddon JM. 1994. Reproducibility of a food frequency questionnaire for use in ocular research. Eye Disease Case-Control Study Group. *Invest Ophthalmol Vis Sci* 35:2725–2733.
Alaimo K, Olson CM, Frongillo EA Jr. 2001a. Food insufficiency and American school-aged children's cognitive, academic, and psychosocial development. *Pediatrics* 108:44–53.
Alaimo K, Olson CM, Frongillo EA Jr. 2001b. Low family income and food insufficiency in relation to overweight in U.S. children: Is there a paradox? *Arch Pediatr Adolesc Med* 155:1161–1167.
Alaimo K, Olson CM, Frongillo EA Jr, Briefel RR. 2001c. Food insufficiency, family income, and health in U.S. preschool and school-aged children. *Am J Public Health* 91:781–786.

Allen KG, Harris MA. 2001. The role of n-3 fatty acids in gestation and parturition. *Exp Biol Med* 226:498–506.

American College of Obstetricians and Gynecologists. 1994. *ACOG Technical Bulletin Number 189: Exercise During Pregnancy and the Postpartum Period*. Washington, DC: ACOG Press.

Andersen RE, Crespo CJ, Bartlett SJ, Cheskin LJ, Pratt M. 1998. Relationship of physical activity and television watching with body weight and level of fatness among children: Results from the Third National Health and Nutrition Examination Survey. *J Am Med Assoc* 279:938–942.

Angus RM, Sambrook PN, Pocock NA, Eisman JA. 1989. A simple method for assessing calcium intake in Caucasian women. *J Am Diet Assoc* 89:209–214.

Bailey RC, Olson J, Pepper SL, Porszasz J, Barstow TJ, Cooper DM. 1995. The level and tempo of children's physical activities: An observational study. *Med Sci Sports Exerc* 27:1033–1041.

Ballew C, Kuester S, Gillespie C. 2000. Beverage choices affect adequacy of children's nutrient intakes. *Arch Pediatr Adolesc Med* 154:1148–1152.

Baranowski T. 1985. Methodologic issues in self-report of health behavior. *J Sch Health* 55:179–182.

Baranowski T. 1988. Validity and reliability of self report measures of physical activity: An information-processing perspective. *Res Q Exerc Sport* 59:314–327.

Baranowski T. 1997a. Families and health action. In: Gochman DS, ed. *Handbook of Health Behavior Research, Vol. IV: Relevance for Professionals and Issues for the Future*. New York: Plenum. Pp. 179–206.

Baranowski T. 1997b. Psychosocial and sociocultural factors that influence nutritional behaviors and interventions: Cardiovascular disease. In: Garza C, Haas J, Habicht J-P, Pelletier D, eds. *Beyond Nutritional Recommendations: Implementing Science for Healthier Populations*. Ithaca, NY: Cornell University. Pp. 163–188.

Baranowski T, de Moor C. 2000. How many days was that? Intra-individual variability and physical activity assessment. *Res Q Exerc Sport* 71:S74–S78.

Baranowski T, Hearn M. 1997. Families and health behavior change. In: Gochman DS, ed. *Handbook of Health Behavior Research, Vol. IV: Relevance for Professionals and Issues for the Future*. New York: Plenum. Pp. 303–323.

Baranowski T, Simons-Morton BG. 1991. Dietary and physical activity assessment in school-aged children: Measurement issues. *J Sch Health* 61:195–197.

Baranowski T, Sprague D, Baranowski J, Harrison J. 1991. Accuracy of maternal dietary recall for preschool children. *J Am Diet Assoc* 91:669–674.

Baranowski T, Bouchard C, Bar-Or O, Bricker T, Heath G, Kimm SYS, Malina R, Obarzanek E, Pate R, Strong WB, Truman B, Washington R. 1992. Assessment, prevalence, and cardiovascular benefits of physical activity and fitness in youth. *Med Sci Sports Exerc* 24:S237–S247.

Baranowski T, Thompson WO, DuRant RH, Baranowski J, Puhl J. 1993. Observations on physical activity in physical locations: Age, gender, ethnicity, and month effects. *Res Q Exerc Sport* 64:127–133.

Baranowski T, Lin LS, Wetter DW, Resnicow K, Hearn MD. 1997. Theory as mediating variables: Why aren't community interventions working as desired? *Ann Epidemiol* 7:S89–S95.

Baranowski T, Anderson C, Carmack C. 1998. Mediating variable framework in physical activity interventions. How are we doing? How might we do better? *Am J Prev Med* 15:266–297.

Baranowski T, Cullen K, Baranowski J. 1999. Psychosocial correlates of dietary intake. *Annu Rev Nutr* 19:17–40.

Baranowski T, Mendlein J, Resnicow K, Frank E, Cullen KW, Baranowski J. 2000. Physical activity and nutrition (PAN) in children and youth: Behavior, genes, and tracking in obesity prevention. *Prev Med* 31:S1–S10.

Baranowski T, Baranowski J, Cullen K. In press. Results of 5 a day achievement badge for African-American Boy Scouts. *Prev Med*.

Barlow SE, Dietz WH. 1998. Obesity evaluation and treatment: Expert committee recommendations. *Pediatrics* 102:E29.

Bartlett S, Brown-Lyons M, Moore D, Estacion A. 2000. *WIC Participant and Program Characteristics 1998*. Alexandria, VA: U.S. Department of Agriculture, Food and Nutrition Service.

Basiotis PP, Welsh SO, Cronin FJ, Kelsay JL, Mertz W. 1987. Number of days of food intake records required to estimate individual and group nutrient intakes with defined confidence. *J Nutr* 117:1638–1641.

Baughcum AE, Chamberlin LA, Deeks CM, Powers SW, Whitaker RC. 2000. Maternal perceptions of overweight preschool children. *Pediatrics* 106:1380–1386.

Baxter SD, Thompson WO, Davis HC, Johnson MH. 1997. Impact of gender, ethnicity, meal component, and time interval between eating and reporting on accuracy of fourth-graders' self-reports of school lunch. *J Am Diet Assoc* 97:1293–1298.

Beaton GH. 1994. Approaches to analysis of dietary data: Relationship between planned analyses and choice of methodology. *Am J Clin Nutr* 59:253S–261S.

Berenson GS, McMahan CA, Voors AW, Webber LS, Srinivasan SR, Frank GC, Foster TA, Blonde CV. 1980. *Cardiovascular Risk Factors in Children: The Early Natural History of Atherosclerosis and Essential Hypertension*. New York: Oxford University Press.

Bild DE, Jacobs DR Jr, Sidney S, Haskell WL, Anderssen N, Oberman A. 1993. Physical activity in young black and white women. The CARDIA Study. *Ann Epidemiol* 3:636–644.

Bingham SA. 1987. The dietary assessment of individuals: Methods, accuracy, new techniques, and recommendations. *Nutr Abstr Rev* 57:705–742.

Bingham SA. 1991. Limitations of the various methods for collecting dietary intake data. *Ann Nut Metab Basel* 35:117–127.

Black MM. 1999. Feeding problems: An ecological perspective. *J Pediatr Psych* 24:217–219.

Block G, Abrams B. 1993. Vitamin and mineral status of women of childbearing potential. *Ann N Y Acad Sci* 678:244–254.

Block G, Clifford C, Naughton DM, Henderson M, McAdams M. 1989. A brief dietary screen for high-fat intake. *J Nutr Educ* 21:199–207.

Block G, Hartman AM, Naughton D. 1990. A reduced dietary questionnaire: Development and validation. *Epidemiology* 1:58–64.

Blum RE, Wei EK, Rockett HR, Langeliers JD, Leppert J, Gardner JD, Colditz GA. 1999. Validation of a food frequency questionnaire in native American and Caucasian children 1 to 5 years of age. *Matern Child Health J* 3:167–172.

Blumberg SJ, Bialostosky K, Hamilton WL, Briefel R. 1999. The effectiveness of a short form of the household food security scale. *Am J Public Health* 89:1231–1234.

Bohlscheid-Thomas S, Hoting I, Boeing H, Wahrendorf J. 1997. Reproducibility and relative validity of energy and macronutrient intake of a food frequency questionnaire developed for the German part of the EPIC project. European Prospective Investigation into Cancer and Nutrition. *Int J Epidemiol* 26:S71–S81.

Bowman SA, Lino M, Gerrior SA, Basiotis PP. 1998. *The Healthy Eating Index, 1994–96*. Washington, DC: U.S. Department of Agriculture, Center for Nutrition Policy and Promotion.

Briefel RR, Flegal KM, Winn DM, Loria CM, Johnson CL, Sempos CT. 1992. Assessing the nation's diet: Limitations of the food frequency questionnaire. *J Am Diet Assoc* 92:959–962.

Briefel RR, McDowell MA, Alaimo K, Caughman CR, Bischof AL, Caroll MD, Johnson CL. 1995. Total energy intake of the U.S. population: The Third National Health and Nutrition Examination Survey, 1988–1991. *Am J Clin Nutr* 62:1072S–1080S.

Briefel RR, Sempos CT, McDowell MA, Chien S, Alaimo K. 1997. Dietary methods research in the Third National Health and Nutrition Examination Survey: Underreporting of energy intake. *Am J Clin Nutr* 65:1203S–1209S.

Bronfenbrenner U. 1993. The ecology of cognitive development: Research models and fugitive findings. In: Wozniak RH, Fischer KW, eds.

Development in Context: Acting and Thinking in Specific Environments. Hillsdale, NJ: Lawrence Erlbaum Associates.

Brooks-Gunn J, Duncan GJ. 1997. The effects of poverty on children. *Future Child* 7:55–71.

Brown JE, Buzzard IM, Jacobs DR Jr, Hannan PJ, Kushi LH, Barosso GM, Schmid LA. 1996. A food frequency questionnaire can detect pregnancy-related changes in diet. *J Am Diet Assoc* 96:262–266.

Bueno de Mesquita HB, Maisonneuve P, Moerman CJ, Runia S, Boyle P. 1992. Lifetime consumption of alcoholic beverages, tea and coffee and exocrine carcinoma of the pancreas: A population-based case-control study in The Netherlands. *Int J Cancer* 50:514–522.

Bundred P, Kitchiner D, Buchan I. 2001. Prevalence of overweight and obese children between 1989 and 1998: Population-based series of cross-sectional studies. *Br Med J* 322:326.

Burke BS. 1947. The dietary history as a tool in research. *J Am Diet Assoc* 23:1041–1046.

Byers T, Marshall J, Fiedler R, Zielezny M, Graham S. 1985. Assessing nutrient intake with an abbreviated dietary interview. *Am J Epidemiol* 122:41–50.

Byrne C, Ursin G, Ziegler RG. 1996. A comparison of food habit and food frequency data as predictors of breast cancer in the NHANES I/NHEFS cohort. *J Nutr* 126:2757–2764.

Caan B, Horgen DM, Margen S, King JC, Jewell NP. 1987. Benefits associated with WIC supplemental feeding during the interpregnancy interval. *Am J Clin Nutr* 45:29–41.

Caan B, Coates A, Schaffer D. 1995. Variations in sensitivity, specificity, and predictive value of a dietary fat screener modified from Block et al. *J Am Diet Assoc* 95:564–568.

Campbell C, Desjardins E. 1989. A model and research approach for studying the management of limited food resources by low-income families. *J Nutr Educ* 21:162–171.

Carleson S, Briefel R. 1995. The USDA and NHANES food sufficiency questions as an indicator of hunger and food insecurity. In: *Conference on Food Security Measurement and Research: Papers and Proceedings.* Alexandria, VA: U.S. Deparment of Agriculture, Food and Consumer Services. Pp. 48–56.

Carriquiry AL. 1999. Assessing the prevalence of nutrient inadequacy. *Public Health Nutr* 2:23–33.

Casey PH, Szeto K, Lensing S, Bogle M, Weber J. 2001. Children in food-insufficient, low-income families. *Arch Pediatr Adolesc Med* 155:508–514.

CDC (Centers for Disease Control and Prevention). 1996. Nutritional status of children participating in the Special Supplemental Nutrition Program for

Women, Infants, and Children—United States, 1988–1991. *Morb Mortal Wkly Rep* 45:65–69.

CDC 1998a. *Pediatric Nutrition Surveillance, 1997 Full Report.* Atlanta: U.S. Department of Health and Human Services, CDC.

CDC. 1998b. Recommendations to prevent and control iron deficiency in the United States. *Morb Mortal Wkly Rep* 47:1–29.

CDC. 2001. *Behavioral Risk Factor Surveillance System.* Online. National Center for Chronic Disease Prevention and Health Promotion. Available at www.cdc.gov/nccdphp/brfss/. Accessed December 31, 2001.

Certain LK, Kahn RS. 2001. Social gradients in television viewing among very young children. *Pediatr Res* 49:17a.

Clapp JF 3rd. 2000. Exercise during pregnancy. A clinical update. *Clin Sports Med* 19:273–286.

Clemens LHE, Slawson DL, Klesges RC. 1999. The effect of eating out on quality of diet in premenopausal women. *J Am Diet Assoc* 99:442–444.

Cleveland LE, Cook DA, Krebs-Smith S, Friday J. 1997. Method for assessing food intakes in terms of servings based on food guidance. *Am J Clin Nutr* 65:1254S–1263S.

Cnattingius S, Bergstrom R, Lipworth L, Kramer MS. 1998. Prepregnancy weight and the risk of adverse pregnancy outcomes. *N Engl J Med* 338:191–192.

CNPP (Center for Nutrition Policy and Promotion). 1999. *Tips for Using the Food Guide Pyramid for Young Children 2 to 6 Years Old.* Washington, DC: U.S. Department of Agriculture.

Colditz GA, Willett WC, Stampfer MJ, Sampson L, Rosner B, Hennekens CH, Speizer FE. 1987. The influence of age, relative weight, smoking, and alcohol intake on the reproducibility of a dietary questionnaire. *Int J Epidemiol* 16:392–398.

Coon KA, Goldberg J, Rogers BL, Tucker KL. 2001. Relationships between use of television during meals and children's food consumption patterns. *Pediatrics* 107:E7.

Costanzo PR, Woody EZ. 1984. Parental perspectives on obesity in children: The importance of sex differences. *J Social Clin Psychol* 2:305–313.

Crawford DA, Jeffery RW, French SA. 1999. Television viewing, physical inactivity and obesity. *Int J Obes Relat Metab Disord* 23:437–440.

Cronin FJ. 1987. Developing a food guidance system to implement the dietary guidelines. *J Nutr Educ* 19:281–302.

Davis CA, Escobar A, Marcoe KL, Tarone C, Shaw A, Saltos E, Powell R. 1999. *Food Guide Pyramid for Young Children 2 to 6 Years Old: Technical Report on Background and Development.* Washington, DC: U.S. Department of Agriculture, Center for Nutrition Policy and Promotion.

Derrickson JP, Fisher AG, Anderson JEL, Brown AC. 2001. An assessment of various household food security measures in Hawaii has implications for national food security research and monitoring. *J Nutr* 131:749–757.

Dietary Guidelines Advisory Committee. 2000. *Report of the Dietary Guidelines Advisory Committee on the Dietary Guidelines for Americans, 2000.* Washington, DC: U.S. Department of Agriculture, Agricultural Research Service.

Dietz WH, Gortmaker SL. 1985. Do we fatten our children at the television set? Obesity and television viewing in children and adolescents. *Pediatrics* 75:807–812.

Domel S, Baranowski T, Davis H, Leonard SB, Riley P, Baranowski J. 1994. Fruit and vegetable food frequencies by fourth and fifth grade students: Validity and reliability. *J Am Coll Nutr* 13:1–7.

Donovan UM, Gibson RS. 1996. Dietary intakes of adolescent females consuming vegetarian, semi-vegetarian, and omnivorous diets. *J Adolesc Health* 18:292–300.

DuRant RH, Baranowski T, Johnson M, Thompson WO. 1994. The relationship among television watching, physical activity, and body composition of young children. *Pediatrics* 94:449–455.

Dutta MJ, Youn S. 1999. Profiling healthy eating consumers: A psychographic approach to social marketing. *Soc Mark Q* 5:5–21.

Dwyer JT. 1999. Dietary assessment. In: Shils ME, Olson JA, Shike M, Ross AC, eds. *Modern Nutrition in Health and Disease*, 9th ed. Baltimore: Williams and Wilkins. Pp. 937–959.

Edmonds J, Baranowski T, Baranowski J, Cullen KW, Myres D. 2001. Ecological and socioeconomic correlates of fruit and vegetable consumption among children. *Prev Med* 32:476–481.

EPIC Group of Spain. 1997. Relative validity and reproducibility of a diet history questionnaire in Spain. III. Biochemical markers. *Int J Epidemiol* 26:S110–S117.

Eyler AA, Baker E, Cromer L, King AC, Brownson RC, Donatelle RJ. 1998. Physical activity and minority women: A qualitative study. *Health Educ Behav* 25:640–652.

Fagot-Campagna A, Pettitt DJ, Engelgau MM, Burrows NR, Geiss LS, Valdez R, Beckles GLA, Saaddine J, Gregg EW, Williamson DF, Narayan KMV. 2000. Type 2 diabetes among North American children and adolescents: An epidemiologic review and a public health perspective. *J Pediatr* 136:664–672.

Feskanich D, Rimm EB, Giovannucci EL, Colditz GA, Stampfer MJ, Litin LB, Willett WC. 1993. Reproducibility and validity of food intake measurements from a semiquantitative food frequency questionnaire. *J Am Diet Assoc* 93:790–796.

Field AE, Colditz GA, Fox MK, Byers T, Serdula M, Bosch RJ, Peterson KE. 1998. Comparison of 4 questionnaires for assessment of fruit and vegetable intake. *Am J Public Health* 88:1216–1218.

Flegal KM, Carroll RJ, Kuczmarski RJ, Johnson CL. 1998. Overweight and obesity in the United States: Prevalence and trends, 1960–1994. *Int J Obes Relat Metab Disord* 22:39–47.

FNS (Food and Nutrition Service). 1998. *WIC Policy Memorandum 98-9. Nutrition Risk Criteria.* U.S. Department of Agriculture, Alexandria, VA. June 29.

Ford ES, Merritt RK, Heath GW, Powell KE, Washburn RA, Kriska A, Haile G. 1991. Physical activity behaviors in lower and higher socioeconomic status populations. *Am J Epidemiol* 133:1246–1256.

Forshee RA, Storey ML. 2001. The role of added sugars in the diet quality of children and adolescents. *J Am Coll Nutr* 20:32–43.

Fox MK, Burstein N, Golay J, Price C. 1998. *WIC Nutrition Education Assessment Study: Final Report.* Cambridge, MA: Abt Associates Inc.

Frank GC, Nicklas TA, Webber LS, Major C, Miller JF, Berenson GS. 1992. A food frequency questionnaire for adolescents: Defining eating patterns. *J Am Diet Assoc* 92:313–318.

Freedman DS, Dietz WH, Srinivasan SR, Berenson GS. 1999. The relation of overweight to cardiovascular risk factors among children and adolescents: The Bogalusa Heart Study. *Pediatrics* 103:1175–1182.

Freedson PS, Miller K. 2000. Objective monitoring of physical activity using motion sensors and heart rate. *Res Q Exerc Sport* 71:21–29.

Freeman, Sullivan & Co. 1994. *WIC Dietary Assessment Validation Study. Final Report.* San Francisco: Freeman, Sullivan & Co.

French SA, Harnack L, Jeffery RW. 2000. Fast food restaurant use among women in the Pound of Prevention study: Dietary, behavioural, and demographic correlates. *Int J Obes Relat Metab Disord* 24:1353–1359.

Friis S, Kruger Kjaer S, Stripp C, Overvad K. 1997. Reproducibility and relative validity of a self-administered semiquantitative food frequency questionnaire applied to younger women. *J Clin Epidemiol* 50:303–311.

Fung TT, Rimm EB, Spiegelman D, Rifai N, Tofler GH, Willett WC, Hu FB. 2001. Association between dietary patterns and plasma biomarkers of obesity and cardiovascular disease risk. *Am J Clin Nutr* 73:61–67.

Galtier-Dereure F, Montpeyroux F, Boulot P, Bringer J, Jaffiol C. 1995. Weight excess before pregnancy: Complications and cost. *Int J Obes Relat Metab Disord* 19:443–448.

Galtier-Dereure F, Boegner C, Bringer J. 2000. Obesity and pregnancy: Complications and cost. *Am J Clin Nutr* 71:1242S–1248S.

Garcia AW, Broda MA, Frenn M, Coviak C, Pender NJ, Ronis DL. 1995. Gender and developmental differences in exercise beliefs among youth and prediction of their exercise behavior. *J Sch Health* 65:213–219.

Gardner JD, Suitor CJ, Witschi J, Wang Q. 1991. *Dietary Assessment Methodology for Use in the Special Supplemental Food Program for Women, Infants and Children (WIC)*. Boston: Harvard School of Public Health.

Gillman MW, Rifas-Shiman SL, Frazier AL, Rockett HR, Camargo CA Jr, Field AE, Berkey CS, Colditz GA. 2000. Family dinner and diet quality among older children and adolescents. *Arch Fam Med* 9:235–240.

Glanz K, Maibach E, Basil M, Goldberg J, Snyder D. 1998. Why Americans eat what they do: Taste, nutrition, cost, convenience and weight control concerns as influences on food consumption. *J Am Diet Assoc* 98:1118–1126.

Gleason P, Rangarajan A, Olson C. 2000. *Dietary Intake and Dietary Attitudes Among Food Stamp Participants and Other Low-Income Individuals*. Princeton, NJ: Mathematica Policy Research.

Goldenberg RL, Tamura T, Neggers Y, Copper RL, Johnston KE, DuBard MB, Hauth JC. 1995. The effect of zinc supplementation on pregnancy outcome. *J Am Med Assoc* 274:463–468.

Goran MI. 1998. Measurement issues related to studies of childhood obesity: Assessment of body composition, body fat distribution, physical activity, and food intake. *Pediatrics* 101:S505–S518.

Goran MI, Gower BA, Nagy TR, Johnson RK. 1998. Developmental changes in energy expenditure and physical activity in children: Evidence for a decline in physical activity in girls before puberty. *Pediatrics* 101:887–891.

Gordon-Larsen P, McMurray RG, Popkin BM. 1999. Adolescent physical activity and inactivity vary by ethnicity: The National Longitudinal Study of Adolescent Health. *J Pediatr* 135:301–306.

Gorman K. 1995. Malnutrition and cognitive development: Evidence from experimental/quasi-experimental studies among the mild-to-moderately malnourished. *J Nutr* 125:2239S–2244S.

Gorn GJ, Goldberg ME. 1982. Behavioral evidence for the effects of televised food messages on children's diet and physical activity. *J Consum Res* 9:200–205.

Gortmaker S, Must A, Sobol A, Peterson K, Colditz G, Dietz W. 1996. Television viewing as a cause of increasing obesity among children in the United States, 1986–1990. *Arch Pediatr Adolesc Med* 150:356–362.

Grantham-McGregor S, Ani C. 2001. A review of studies on the effect of iron deficiency on cognitive development in children. *J Nutr* 131:649S–666S.

Guillame M, Lapidus L, Beckers F, Lamber A, Bjorntorp P. 1995. Familial trends of obesity through three generations: The Belgian-Luxembourg Child Study. *Int J Obes Relat Metab Disord* 19:S5–S9.

Gunderson EP, Abrams B, Selvin S. 2000. The relative importance of gestational gain and maternal characteristics associated with the risk of becoming overweight after pregnancy. *Int J Obes Relat Metab Disord* 24:1660–1668.

Haile RW, Hunt IF, Buckley J, Browdy BL, Murphy NJ, Alpers D. 1986. Identifying a limited number of foods important in supplying selected dietary nutrients. *J Am Diet Assoc* 86:611–616.

Harro M. 1997. Validation of a questionnaire to assess physical activity of children ages 4–8 years. *Res Q Exerc Sport* 68:259–268.

Haste FM, Brooke OG, Anderson HR, Bland JM, Shaw A, Griffin J, Peacock JL. 1990. Nutrient intakes during pregnancy: Observations on the influence of smoking and social class. *Am J Clin Nutr* 51:29–36.

Hearn M, Baranowski T, Baranowski J, et al. 1998. Environmental influences on dietary behavior among children: Availability and accessibility of fruits and vegetables enable consumption. *J Health Educ* 29:26–32.

Hebert JR, Miller DR. 1991. The inappropriateness of conventional use of the correlation coefficient in assessing validity and reliability of dietary assessment methods. *Eur J Epidemiol* 7:339–343.

HHS (Department of Health and Human Services). 1996. *Physical Activity and Health: A Report of the Surgeon General*. Atlanta: Centers for Disease Control and Prevention, National Center for Chronic Disease Prevention and Health Promotion.

HHS. 2000. *Healthy People 2010*. 2nd ed. Washington DC: U.S. Government Printing Office.

Huijbregts PP, Feskens EJ, Kromhout D. 1995. Dietary patterns and cardiovascular risk factors in elderly men: The Zutphen Elderly Study. *Int J Epidemiol* 24:313–320.

Hunter DJ, Sampson L, Stampfer MJ, Colditz GA, Rosner B, Willett WC. 1988. Variability in portion sizes of commonly consumed foods among a population of women in the United States. *Am J Epidemiol* 127:1240–1249.

Hupkens CLH, Knibble RA, Drop MJ. 1997. Social class differences in women's fat and fibre consumption: A cross-national study. *Appetite* 28:131–149.

Innis SM. 2000. The role of dietary n-6 and n-3 fatty acids in the developing brain. *Dev Neurosci* 22:474–480.

IOM (Institute of Medicine). 1990. *Nutrition During Pregnancy*. Washington, DC: National Academy Press.

IOM. 1996. *WIC Nutrition Risk Criteria: A Scientific Assessment*. Washington, DC: National Academy Press.

IOM. 1997. *Dietary Reference Intakes for Calcium, Phosphorus, Magnesium, Vitamin D, and Fluoride*. Washington, DC: National Academy Press.

IOM. 1998. *Dietary Reference Intakes for Thiamin, Riboflavin, Niacin, Vitamin B_6, Folate, Vitamin B_{12}, Pantothenic Acid, Biotin, and Choline.* Washington, DC: National Academy Press.

IOM. 2000a. *Dietary Reference Intakes: Applications in Dietary Assessment.* Washington DC: National Academy Press.

IOM. 2000b. *Dietary Reference Intakes for Vitamin C, Vitamin E, Selenium, and Carotenoids.* Washington, DC: National Academy Press.

IOM. 2000c. *Framework for Dietary Risk Assessment in the WIC Program: An Interim Report.* Washington DC: National Academy Press.

IOM. 2001. *Dietary Reference Intakes for Vitamin A, Vitamin K, Arsenic, Boron, Chromium, Copper, Iodine, Iron, Manganese, Molybdenum, Nickel, Silicon, Vanadium, and Zinc.* Washington, DC: National Academy Press.

Jacobs C, Dwyer JT. 1988. Vegetarian children: Appropriate and inappropriate diets. *Am J Clin Nutr* 48:S811–S818.

Jacques PF, Tucker KL. 2001. Are dietary patterns useful for understanding the role of diet in chronic disease? *Am J Clin Nutr* 73:1–2.

Jain A, Sherman SN, Chamberlin LA, Carter Y, Powers SW, Whitaker RC. 2001. Why don't low-income mothers worry about their preschoolers being overweight? *Pediatrics* 107:1138–1146.

Jain M, McLaughlin J. 2000. Validity of nutrient estimates by food frequency questionnaires based either on exact frequencies or categories. *Ann Epidemiol* 10:354–360.

Jain M, Howe GR, Rohan T. 1996. Dietary assessment in epidemiology: Comparison on food frequency and a diet history questionnaire with a 7-day food record. *Am J Epidemiol* 143:953–960.

Janelle KC, Barr SI. 1995. Nutrient intakes and eating behavior scores of vegetarian and non-vegetarian women. *J Am Diet Assoc* 95:180–186.

Jarvinen R, Seppanen R, Knekt P. 1993. Short-term and long-term reproducibility of dietary history interview data. *Int J Epidemiol* 22:520–527.

Jeffery RW, French SA. 1998. Epidemic obesity in the United States: Are fast foods and television viewing contributing? *Am J Public Health* 88:277–280.

Jeffrey DB, McLellarn RW, Fox DT. 1982. The development of children's eating habits: The role of television commercials. *Health Educ Q* 9:78–93.

Johnson RK, Soultanakis RP, Matthews DE. 1998. Literacy and body fatness are associated with underreporting of energy intake in U.S. low-income women using the multiple-pass 24-hour recall: A doubly labeled water study. *J Am Diet Assoc* 98:1136–1140.

Kant AK, Schatzkin A, Graubard BI, Schairer C. 2000. A prospective study of diet quality and mortality in women. *J Am Med Assoc* 283:2109–2115.

Karp R, Greene G. 1983. The effect of rising food costs on the occurrence of malnutrition among the poor in the United States: The Engels phenomenon in 1983. *Bull N Y Acad Med* 59:721–727.

Kaskoun MC, Johnson RK, Goran MI. 1994. Comparison of energy intake by semiquantitative food-frequency questionnaire with total energy expenditure by the doubly labeled water method in young children. *Am J Clin Nutr* 60:43–47.

Kendall A, Olson CM, Frongillo EA Jr. 1996. Relationship of hunger and food insecurity to food availability and consumption. *J Am Diet Assoc* 96:1019–1024.

Kennedy E, Goldberg J. 1995. What are American children eating? Implications for public policy. *Nutr Rev* 53:111–126.

Kennedy ET, Ohls J, Carlson S, Fleming K. 1995. The healthy eating index: Design and applications. *J Am Diet Assoc* 95:1103–1108.

Kim I, Hungerford DW, Yip R, Kuester SA, Zyrkowski C, Trowbridge FL. 1992. Pregnancy nutrition surveillance system—United States, 1979–1990. *MMWR CDC Surveill Summ* 41:25–41.

Klesges RC, Eck LH, Hanson CL, Haddock CK, Klesges LM. 1990. Effects of obesity, social interactions, and physical environment on physical activity in preschoolers. *Health Psychol* 9:435–449.

Klesges RC, Eck LH, Ray JW. 1995a. Who underreports dietary intake in a dietary recall? Evidence from the Second National Health and Nutrition Examination Survey. *J Consult Clin Psychol* 63:438–444.

Klesges RC, Klesges LM, Eck LH, Shelton ML. 1995b. A longitudinal analysis of accelerated weight gain in preschool children. *Pediatrics* 95:126–130.

Knol LL, Haughton B. 1998. Fruit and juice intake associated with higher dietary status index in rural east Tennessee women living in public housing. *J Am Diet Assoc* 98:576–599.

Kohl HW, Fulton JE, Caspersen CJ. 2000. Assessment of physical activity among children and adolescents: A review and synthesis. *Prev Med* 31:S54–S76.

Kramer-LeBlanc CS, Mardis A, Gerrior S, Gaston N. 1999. *Review of the Nutritional Status of WIC Participants: Final Report*. Washington, DC: U.S. Department of Agriculture, Center for Nutrition Policy and Promotion.

Kratt P, Reynolds K, Shewchuck R. 2000. The role of availability as a moderator of family fruit and vegetable consumption. *Health Educ Behav* 27:471–482.

Krebs-Smith SM, Cleveland LE, Ballard-Barbash R, Cook DA, Kahle LL. 1997. Characterizing food intake patterns of American adults. *Am J Clin Nutr* 65:1264S–1268S.

Kriska AM, Caspersen CJ. 1997. A collection of physical activity questionnaires for health-related research. *Med Sci Sports Exerc* 29:S1–S205.

Kristal AR, Shattuck AL, Henry HJ. 1990. Patterns of dietary behavior associated with selecting diets low in fat: Reliability and validity of a behavioral approach to dietary assessment. *J Am Diet Assoc* 90:214–220.

Kroke A, Klipstein-Grobusch K, Voss S, Moseneder J, Thielecke F, Noack R, Boeing H. 1999. Validation of a self-administered food-frequency questionnaire administered in the European Prospective Investigation into Cancer and Nutrition (EPIC) Study: Comparison of energy, protein, and macronutrient intakes estimated with the doubly labeled water, urinary nitrogen, and repeated 24-h dietary recall methods. *Am J Clin Nutr* 70:439–474.

Kuczmarski RJ, Flegal KM, Campbell SM, Johnson CL. 1994. Increasing prevalence of overweight among U.S. adults: National Health and Nutrition Examination Surveys, 1960 to 1991. *J Am Med Assoc* 272:205–211.

Kuczmarski RJ, Carroll MD, Flegal KM, Troiano RP. 1997. Varying body mass index cutoff points to describe overweight prevalence among U.S. adults: NHANES III (1988 to 1994). *Obes Res* 5:542–548.

Kuczmarski RJ, Ogden CL, Grummer-Strawn LM, Flegal KM, Guo SS, Wei R, Mei Z, Curtin LR, Roche AF, Johnson CL. 2000. CDC growth charts: United States. *Adv Data* 8:1–27.

Lee JS, Fongillo EA Jr. 2001. Understanding need is important for assessing the impact of food assistance program participation on nutritional and health status in U.S. elderly persons. *J Nutr* 131:765–773.

Levitsky DA, Strupp BJ. 1995. Malnutrition and the brain: Changing concepts, changing concerns. *J Nutr* 125:2212S–2220S.

Liu K. 1994. Statistical issues related to semiquantitative food-frequency questionnaires. *Am J Clin Nutr* 59:262S–265S.

Longnecker MP, Lissner L, Holden JM, Flack VF, Taylor PR, Stampfer MJ, Willett WC. 1993. The reproducibility and validity of a self-administered semiquantitative food frequency questionnaire in subjects from South Dakota and Wyoming. *Epidemiology* 4:356–365.

Looker AC, Dallman PR, Carroll MD, Gunter EW, Johnson CL. 1997. Prevalence of iron deficiency in the United States. *J Am Med Assoc* 277:973–976.

LSRO/FASEB (Life Sciences Research Office/Federation of American Societies for Experimental Biology). 1995. *Third Report on Nutrition Monitoring in the United States*. Vols. 1 and 2. Washington DC: U.S. Government Printing Office.

Ma J, Betts NM, Hampl JS. 2000. Clustering of lifestyle behaviors: The relationship between cigarette smoking, alcohol consumption, and dietary intake. *Am J Health Promot* 15:107–117.

Ma J, Betts NM, Hampl JS. Certain LK, Kahn RS. 2001. Social gradients in television viewing among very young children. *Pediatr Res* 49:17a.

Macera CA, Pratt M. 2000. Public health surveillance of physical activity. *Res Q Exerc Sport* 71:97–103.

Manios Y, Kafatos A, Markakis G. 1998. Physical activity in 6-year-old children: Validation of two proxy reports. *Pediatr Exerc Sci* 10:176–188.

Mardis AL, Anand R. 2000. A look at the diet of pregnant women. *Nutrition Insights 17*. Washington, DC: U.S. Department of Agriculture, Center for Nutrition Policy and Promotion.

Masse LC, Ainsworth BE, Tortolero S, Levin S, Fulton JE, Henderson KA, Mayo K. 1998. Measuring physical activity in midlife, older, and minority women: Issues from an expert panel. *J Womens Health* 7:57–67.

Matthews CE, Hebert JR, Ockene IS, Saperia G, Merriam PA. 1997. Relationship between leisure time physical activity and selected dietary variables in the Worcester Area Trial for Counseling in Hyperlipidemia. *Med Sci Sports Exerc* 29:1199–1207.

McCann SE, Trevisan M, Priore RL, Muti P, Markovic N, Russell M, Chan AW, Freudenheim JL. 1999. Comparability of nutrient estimation by three food frequency questionnaires for use in epidemiological studies. *Nutr Cancer* 35:4–9.

McCrory MA, Fuss PJ, Hays NP, Vinken AG, Greenberg AS, Roberts SB. 1999. Overeating in America: Association between restaurant food consumption and body fatness in healthy adult men and women ages 19 to 80. *Obes Res* 7:564–571.

McCullough ML, Feskanich D, Stampfer MJ, Rosner BA, Hu FB, Hunter DJ, Variyam JN, Colditz GA, Willett WC. 2000. Adherence to the Dietary Guidelines for Americans and risk of major chronic disease in women. *Am J Clin Nutr* 72:1214–1222.

McPherson RS, Hoelscher DM, Alexander M, Scanlon KS, Serdula MK. 2000. Dietary assessment methods among school-aged children: Validity and reliability. *Prev Med* 31:S11–S33.

Mei Z, Scanlon KS, Grummer-Strawn LM, Freedman DS, Yip R, Trowbridge FL. 1998. Increasing prevalence of overweight among U.S. low-income preschool children: The Centers for Disease Control and Prevention pediatric nutrition surveillance, 1983 to 1995. *Pediatrics* 101:E12.

Millen BE, Quatromoni PA, Copenhafer DL, Demistic S, O'Horo CE, D'Agostino RB. 2001. Validation of a dietary pattern approach for evaluating nutritional risk: The Framingham Nutrition Studies. *J Am Diet Assoc* 101:187–194.

Mokdad AH, Serdula MK, Dietz WH, Bowman BA, Marks JS, Koplan JP. 1999. The spread of the obesity epidemic in the United States, 1991–1998. *J Am Med Assoc* 282:1519–1522.

Mokdad AH, Ford ES, Bowman BA, Nelson DE, Engelgau MM, Vinicor F, Marks JS. 2000. Diabetes trends in the US: 1990–1998. *Diabetes Care* 23:1278–1283.

Mori TA, Beilin LJ. 2001. Long-chain omega 3 fatty acids, blood lipids and cardiovascular risk reduction. *Curr Opin Lipidol* 12:11–17.

Munoz KA, Krebs-Smith SM, Ballard-Barbash R, Cleveland LE. 1997. Food intakes of U.S. children and adolescents compared with recommendations. *Pediatrics* 100:323–329.

Must A, Spanado J, Coakley EH, Field AE, Colditz G, Dietz WH. 1999. The disease burden associated with overweight and obesity. *J Am Med Assoc* 282:1523–1529.

Naeye RL. 1990. Maternal body weight and pregnancy outcome. *Am J Clin Nutr* 5:273–279.

NCHS (National Center for Health Statistics). 1994. *Conference on Food Security Measurement and Research: Papers and proceedings*, January 21–22, 1994, Washington, DC. Hyattsville, MD: NCHS.

NCHS. 1998. *Health, United States, 1998 with Socioeconomic Status and Health Chartbook*. Hyattsville, MD: NCHS.

Negri E, Franceschi S, La Vecchia C, Filiberti R, Guarneri S, Nanni O, Decarli A. 1994. The application of different correlation coefficients to assess the reproducibility of a food frequency questionnaire. *Eur J Cancer Prev* 3:489–497.

Nelson M, Black AE, Morris JA, Cole TJ. 1989. Between- and within-subject variation in nutrient intake from infancy to old age: Estimating the number of days required to rank dietary intakes with desired precision. *Am J Clin Nutr* 50:155–167.

Nicklas TA, Myers L, Reger C, Beech B, Berenson GA. 1998. Impact of breakfast consumption on nutritional adequacy of diets of young adults in Bogalusa, Louisiana: Ethnic and gender contrasts. *J Am Diet Assoc* 98:1432–1438.

Nicklas TA, Baranowski T, Baranowski JC, Cullen K, Rittenberry L, Olvera N. 2001. Family and child-care provider influences on preschool children's fruit, juice, and vegetable consumption. *Nutr Rev* 59:224-235.

Nicklas TA, McQuarrie A, Fastnaught DL, O'Neil CE. In press. Efficiency of breakfast consumption patterns of ninth graders: Nutrient-to-cost comparisons. *J Am Diet Assoc*.

NIH (National Institutes of Health). 1998. *Clinical Guidelines on the Identification, Evaluation, and Treatment of Overweight and Obesity in Adults: The Evidence Report*. NIH Publication No. 98-4083. Bethesda, MD: NIH.

NIH Technology Assessment Conference Panel. 1993. Methods for voluntary weight loss and control. *Ann Intern Med* 119:764–770.

NRC (National Research Council). 1989. *Recommended Dietary Allowances*. 10th ed. Washington DC: National Academy Press.

Nusser SM, Carriquiry AL, Dodd KW, Fuller WA. 1996. A semiparametric transformation approach to estimating usual daily intake distributions. *J Am Stat Assoc* 91:1440–1449.

Ogden CL, Troiano RP, Briefel RR, Kuczmarski RJ, Flegal KM, Johnson CL. 1997. Prevalence of overweight among preschool children in the United States, 1971 through 1994. *Pediatrics* 99:E1–E12.

Olson CM. 1999. Nutrition and health outcomes associated with food insecurity and hunger. *J Nutr* 129:521–524.

Pao EM, Cypel YS. 1996. Estimation of dietary intake. In: Ziegler EE, Filer LJ Jr, eds. *Present Knowledge in Nutrition*. Washington, DC: ILSI Press. Pp. 498–507.

Pate RR. 1993. Physical activity assessment in children and adolescents. *Crit Rev Food Sci Nutr* 33:321–326.

Pate RR, Ross JG. 1987. The national children and youth fitness study. II. Factors associated with health-related fitness. *J Phys Educ Recreat Dance* 58:93–95.

Patterson RE, Haines PS, Popkin BM. 1994. Diet quality index: Capturing a multidimensional behavior. *J Am Diet Assoc* 94:57–64.

Pehrsson PR, Moser-Veillon PB, Sims LS, Suitor CW, Russek-Cohen E. 2001. Postpartum iron status in nonlactating participants and nonparticipants in the special supplemental nutrition program for women, infants, and children. *Am J Clin Nutr* 73:86–92.

Persson L, Carlgren G. 1984. Measuring children's diets: Valuation of dietary assessment techniques in infancy and childhood. *Int J Epidemiol* 13:506–517.

Pollitt E. 1988. Developmental impact of nutrition on pregnancy, infancy, and childhood: Public health issues in the United States. *Int Rev Res Ment Retard* 15:33–80.

Power C, Lake JK, Cole TJ. 1997. Measurement and long-term health risks of child and adolescent fatness. *Int J Obes Relat Metab Disord* 21:507–526.

Randall B, Boast L, Holst L. 1995. *Study of WIC Participant and Program Characteristics, 1994*. Cambridge, MA: Abt Associates.

Randall E, Marshall J, Graham S, Brasure J. 1989. Frequency of food use data and the multidimensionality of diet. *J Am Diet Assoc* 89:1070–1075.

Randall E, Marshall JR, Graham S, Brasure J. 1990. Patterns in food use and their associations with nutrient intakes. *Am J Clin Nutr* 52:739–745.

Randall E, Marshall JR, Graham S, Brasure J. 1991a. High-risk health behaviors associated with various dietary patterns. *Nutr Cancer* 16:135–151.

Randall E, Marshall JR, Brasure J, Graham S. 1991b. Patterns in food use and compliance with NCI dietary guidelines. *Nutr Cancer* 15:141–158.

Robinson SK, Godfrey C, Osmond V, Cox, Barker D. 1996. Evaluation of a food frequency questionnaire used to assess nutrient intakes in pregnant women. *Eur J Clin Nutr* 50:302–308.

Robinson TN. 1998. Does television cause obesity? *J Am Med Assoc* 279:959–960.

Robinson TN. 1999. Reducing children's television viewing to prevent obesity. *J Am Med Assoc* 282:1561–1567.

Rockett HRH, Wolf AM, Colditz GA. 1995. Development and reproducibility of a food frequency questionnaire to assess diets of older children and adolescents. *J Am Diet Assoc* 95:336–339.

Rogers MAM, Simon DG, Zucker LB, Mackessy JS, Newman-Palmer MB. 1995. Indicators of poor dietary habits in a high risk population. *J Am Coll Nutr* 14:159–164.

Rosmond R, Baghel F, Holm G, Bjorntorp P. 2000. Gender-related behavior during childhood and associations with adult abdominal obesity: A nested case-control study in women. *J Womens Health Gend Based Med* 9:413–419.

Rowland TW. 1998. The biological basis of physical activity. *Med Sci Sports Exerc* 30:392–399.

Rush D. 1988. The National WIC Evaluation: Evaluation of the Special Supplemental Food Program for Women, Infants and Children. *Am J Clin Nutr* 48:389–519.

Sallis JF, Saelens BE. 2000. Assessment of physical activity by self-report: Status, limitations, and future directions. *Res Q Exerc Sport* 71:S1–S14.

Sallis JF, Nader PR, Broyles SL, Berry CC, Elder JP, McKenzie TL, Nelson JA. 1993. Correlates of physical activity at home in Mexican-American and Anglo-American preschool children. *Health Psychol* 12:390–398.

Sallis JF, McKenzie TL, Elder JP, Broyles SL, Nader PR. 1997. Factors parents use in selecting play spaces for young children. *Arch Pediatr Adolesc Med* 151:414–417.

Sallis JF, Alcaraz JE, McKenzie TL, Hovell MF. 1999. Predictors of change in children's physical activity over 20 months. *Am J Prev Med* 16:222–229.

Sallis JF, Prochaska JJ, Taylor WC. 2000. A review of correlates of physical activity of children and adolescents. *Med Sci Sports Exerc* 32:963–975.

Salvini S, Hunter DJ, Sampson L, Stampfer MJ, Colditz GA, Rosner B, Willett WC. 1989. Food-based validation of a dietary questionnaire: The effects of week-to-week variation in food consumption. *Int J Epidemiol* 18:858–867.

Sampson AE, Dixit S, Meyers AF, Houser R. 1995. The nutritional impact of breakfast consumption on the diets of inner-city African-American elementary school children. *J Natl Med Assoc* 87:195–202.

Sawaya AL, Tucker K, Tsay R, Willett W, Saltzman E, Dallal GE, Roberts SB. 1996. Evaluation of four methods for determining energy intake in young and older women: Comparison with doubly labeled water measurements of total energy expenditure. *Am J Clin Nutr* 63:491–499.

Schaffer DM, Coates AO, Caan BJ, Slattery ML, Potter JD. 1997. Performance of a shortened telephone-administered version of a quantitative food frequency questionnaire. *Ann Epidemiol* 7:463–471.

Schoeller DA. 1990. How accurate is self-reported dietary energy intake? *Nutr Rev* 48:373–379.

Scholl TO, Hediger ML, Schall JI. 1996. Excessive gestational weight gain and chronic disease risk. *Am J Hum Biol* 8:735–741.

Schuette LK, Song WO, Hoerr SL. 1996 Quantitative use of the Food Guide Pyramid to evaluate dietary intake of college students. *J Am Diet Assoc* 96:453–457.

Sempos CT, Johnson NE, Smith EL, Gilligan C. 1985. Effects of intraindividual and interindividual variation in repeated dietary records. *Am J Epidemiol* 121:120–130.

Sempos CT, Briefel RR, Johnson C, Woteki CE. 1992. Process and rationale for selecting dietary methods for NHANES III. *Vital Health Stat 4* 27:85–90.

Sempos CT, Flegal KM, Johnson CL, Loria CM, Woteki CE, Briefel RR. 1993. Issues in the long-term evaluation of diet in longitudinal studies. *J Nutr* 123:406–412.

Serdula MK, Ivery D, Coates RJ, Freedman DS, Williamson DF, Byers T. 1993. Do obese children become obese adults? A review of the literature. *Prev Med* 22:167–177.

Serdula MK, Alexander MP, Scanlon KS, Bowman BA. 2001. What are preschool children eating? A review of dietary assessment. *Annu Rev Nutr* 21:475–498.

Shaw A, Fulton L, Davis C, Hogbin M. 1996. *Using the Food Guide Pyramid: A Resource for Nutrition Educators*. Washington, DC: U.S. Department of Agriculture.

Shaw AE, Escobar AJ, Davis CA. 2000. Reassessing the Food Guide Pyramid: Decision-making framework. *J Nutr Educ* 32:111–118.

Shaw GM, Velie EM, Schaffer D. 1996. Risk of neural tube defect-affected pregnancies among obese women. *J Am Med Assoc* 275:1093–1096.

Sidney S, Sternfeld B, Haskell WL, Jacobs DR Jr, Chesney MA, Hulley SB. 1996. Television viewing and cardiovascular risk factors in young adults: The CARDIA study. *Ann Epidemiol* 6:154–159.

Siega-Riz AM, Carson T, Popkin B. 1998. Three squares or mostly snacks—What do teens really eat? A sociodemographic study of meal patterns. *J Adolesc Health* 22:29–36.

Siega-Riz AM, Popkin BM, Carson T. 2000. Differences in food patterns at breakfast by sociodemographic characteristics among a nationally representative sample of adults in the United States. *Prev Med* 30:415–424.

Sigma One Corporation. 2000. *Nutritional Risk Analysis and Estimation of Eligibility for the Special Supplemental Nutrition Program for Women, Infants, and Children (WIC) in 1989*. Research Triangle Park, NC: Sigma One Corporation.

Slattery ML, Boucher KM, Caan BJ, Potter JD, Ma KN. 1998. Eating patterns and risk of colon cancer. *Am J Epidemiol* 148:4–16.

Smith AF. 1991. Cognitive processes in long-term dietary recall. *Vital Health Stat 6* 4:1–42.

Stein AD, Shea S, Basch CE, Contento IR, Zybert P. 1992. Consistency of the Willett semiquantitative food frequency questionnaire and 24-hour dietary recalls in estimating nutrient intakes of preschool children. *Am J Epidemiol* 135:667–677.

Strauss RS, Burack G, Rodzilsky D, Colin M. In press. Physical activity, self-efficacy, and self-esteem in healthy children. *Arch Pediatr Adolesc Med*.

Strohmeyer SL, Massey LK, Davison MA. 1984. A rapid dietary screening device for clinics. *J Am Diet Assoc* 84:428–432.

Stucky-Ropp RC, DiLorenzo TM. 1993. Determinants of exercise in children. *Prev Med* 22:880–889.

Subar AF, Thompson FE, Smith AF, Jobe JB, Ziegler RG, Potischman N, Schatzkin A, Hartman A, Swanson C, Kruse L. 1995. Improving food frequency questionnaires: A qualitative approach using cognitive interviewing. *J Am Diet Assoc* 95:781–788.

Suitor CJ, Gardner J, Willett WC. 1989. A comparison of food frequency and diet recall methods in studies of nutrient intake of low-income pregnant women. *J Am Diet Assoc* 89:1786–1794.

Suitor CW, Gardner JD, Feldstein ML. 1990. Characteristics of diet among a culturally diverse group of low-income pregnant women. *J Am Diet Assoc* 90:543–549.

Taras HL, Gage M. 1995. Advertised foods on children's television. *Arch Pediatr Adolesc Med* 149:649–652.

Tarasuk V. 1996. Nutritional epidemiology. In: Ziegler EE, Filer LJ Jr, eds. *Present Knowledge in Nutrition*. Washington, DC: ILSI Press. Pp. 508–516.

Tarasuk VS, Beaton GH. 1999. Women's dietary intakes in the context of household food insecurity. *J Nutr* 129:672–679.

Tarasuk VS, Brooker AS. 1997. Interpreting epidemiologic studies of diet-disease relationships. *J Nutr* 127:1847–1852.

Taylor RW, Goulding A. 1998. Validation of a short food frequency questionnaire to assess calcium intake in children aged 3 to 6 years. *Eur J Clin Nutr* 52:464–465.

Thompson FE, Byers T. 1994. Dietary Assessment Resource Manual. *J Nutr* 124:2245S–2317S.

Thompson FE, Kipnis V, Subar AF, Krebs-Smith SM, Kahle LL, Midthune D, Potischman N, Schatzkin A. 2000. Evaluation of 2 brief instruments and a food-frequency questionnaire to estimate daily number of servings of fruit and vegetables. *Am J Clin Nutr* 71:1503–1510.

Toren A, Rechavi G, Ramot B. 1996. Pediatric cancer: Environmental and genetic aspects. *Pediatr Hematol Oncol* 13:319–331.

Townsend MS, Peerson J, Love B, Achterberg C, Murphy SP. 2001. Food insecurity if positively related to overweight in women. *J Nutr* 131:1738–1745.

Tran KM, Johnson RK, Soultanakis RP, Matthews DE. 2000. In-person vs. telephone-administered multiple-pass 24-hour recalls in women: Validation with doubly labeled water. *J Am Diet Assoc* 100:777–783.

Traub RE. 1994. *Reliability for the Social Sciences, Theory and Applications.* Thousand Oaks, CA: Sage.

Treiber FA, Leonard SB, Frank G, Musante L, Davis H, Strong WB, Levy M. 1990. Dietary assessment instruments for preschool children: Reliability of parental responses to the 24-hour recall and a food frequency questionnaire. *J Am Diet Assoc* 90:814–820.

Troiano RP, Briefel RR, Carroll MD, Bialostosky K. 2000. Energy and fat intakes of children and adolescents in the United States: Data from the national examination surveys. *Am J Clin Nutr* 72:1343S–1353S.

Troiano RP, Macera CA, Ballard-Barbash R. 2001. Be physically active each day. How can we know? *J Nutr* 131:451S–460S.

Trost SG, Pate RR, Freedson PS, Sallis JF, Taylor WC. 2000. Using objective physical activity measures with youth: How many days of monitoring are needed? *Med Sci Sports Exerc* 32:426–431.

Tucker KL, Dallal GE, Rush D. 1992. Dietary patterns of elderly Boston-area residents defined by cluster analysis. *J Am Diet Assoc* 92:1487–1491.

Tucker LA, Bagwell M. 1991. Television viewing and obesity in adult females. *Am J Public Health* 81:908–911.

Uauy R, Mena P, Rojas C. 2000. Essential fatty acids in early life: Structural and functional role. *Proc Nutr Soc* 59:3–15.

USDA (U.S. Department of Agriculture). 1992. *The Food Guide Pyramid.* Home and Garden Bulletin No. 252. Washington, DC: U.S. Government Printing Office.

USDA. 2000. *Summary of FY 2000 Food and NSA Grant Levels.* Online. Food and Nutrition Service. Available at: www.fns.usda.gov/wic/programdata/grantsfy2000.htm. Accessed November 14, 2001.

USDA. 2001a. *Food Security in the United States.* Online. Economic Research Service. Available at www.ers.usda.gov/briefing/foodsecurity. Accessed September 17, 2001.

USDA. 2001b. *WIC at a Glance*. Online. Food and Nutrition Service. Available at www.fns.usda.gov/wic/CONTENT/wicataglance.htm. Accessed November 14, 2001.

USDA. 2001c. *WIC Eligibility Requirements*. Online. Food and Nutrition Service. Available at: www.fns.usda.gov/wic/CONTENT/howtoapply/eligibilityrequirements.htm. Accessed November 14, 2001.

USDA. 2001d. *WIC Program: Total Participation*. Online. Food and Nutrition Service. Available at www.fns.usda.gov/pd/wilatest.htm. Accessed November 14, 2001.

USDA/HHS (U.S. Department of Agriculture/U.S. Department of Health and Human Services). 1995. *Nutrition and Your Health: Dietary Guidelines for Americans*, 4th ed. Home and Garden Bulletin No. 232. Washington, DC: U.S. Government Printing Office.

USDA/HHS. 2000. *Nutrition and Your Health: Dietary Guidelines for Americans*, 5th ed. Home and Garden Bulletin No. 232. Washington, DC: U.S. Government Printing Office.

Variyam JN, Blaylock J, Smallwood D. 1998. *USDA's Healthy Eating Index and Nutrition Information*. Technical Bulletin No. 1866. Washington, DC: U.S. Department of Agriculture.

Walker AM, Blettner M. 1985. Comparing imperfect measures of exposure. *Am J Epidemiol* 121:783–790.

Waller DK, Mills JL, Simpson JL, Cunningham GC, Conley MR, Lassman MR, Rhoads GG. 1994. Are obese women at higher risk for producing malformed offspring? *Am J Obstet Gynecol* 170:541–548.

Washburn RA, Heath GW, Jackson AW. 2000. Reliability and validity issues concerning large-scale surveillance of physical activity. *Res Q Exerc Sport* 71:S104–S113.

Wei EK, Gardner J, Field AE, Rosner BA, Colditz GA, Suitor CW. 1999. Validity of a food frequency questionnaire in assessing nutrient intakes of low-income pregnant women. *Matern Child Health J* 4:241–246.

Welk GJ, Wood K. 2000. Physical activity assessments in physical education. *J Phys Educ Recreat Dance* 71:30–40.

Welk GJ, Corbin CB, Dale D. 2000. Measurement issues in the assessment of physical activity in children. *Res Q Exerc Sport* 71:S59–S73.

Welsh SO, Davis C, Shaw A. 1993. *USDA's Food Guide. Background and Development*. Miscellaneous Publication No. 1514. Hyattsville, MD: U.S. Department of Agriculture.

Werler MM, Louik C, Shapiro S, Mitchell AA. 1996. Prepregnant weight in relation to risk of neural tube defects. *J Am Med Assoc* 275:1089–1092.

Whitaker RC, Wright JA, Pepe MS, Seidel KD, Dietz WH. 1997. Predicting obesity in young adulthood from childhood and parental obesity. *N Engl J Med* 337:869–873.

Whitaker RC, Chen B, Chamberlin LA. 2001. Predicting childhood obesity at birth. *Pediatr Res* 40:99A.

White CC, Powell KE, Hogelin GC, Gentry EM, Forman MR. 1987. The behavioral risk factor surveys. IV. The descriptive epidemiology of exercise. *Am J Prev Med* 3:304–310.

WHO (World Health Organization). 1995. *Physical Status: The Use and Interpretation of Anthropometry*. WHO Technical Report Series, No. 854. Geneva: WHO.

Willett WC. 2000. Accuracy of food-frequency questionnaires. *Am J Clin Nutr* 72:1234–1236.

Willett WC, Reynolds RD, Cottrell-Hoehner S, Sampson L, Browne ML. 1987. Validation of a semi-quantitative food frequency questionnaire: Comparison with a 1-year diet record. *J Am Diet Assoc* 87:43–47.

Windsor R, Baranowski T, Clark N, Cutter G. 1994. *Evaluation of Health Promotion, Health Education, and Disease Prevention Programs*. 2nd ed. Mountain View, CA: Mayfield Publishing.

Wirfalt AKE, Jeffery RW. 1997. Using cluster analysis to examine dietary patterns: Nutrient intakes, gender, and weight status differ across food pattern clusters. *J Am Diet Assoc* 97:272–279.

Wirfalt AK, Jeffery RW, Elmer PJ. 1998. Comparison of food frequency questionnaires: The reduced Block and Willett questionnaires differ in ranking on nutrient intakes. *Am J Epidemiol* 148:1148–1156.

Wolff CB, Wolff HK. 1995. Maternal eating patterns and birth weight of Mexican American infants. *Nutr Health* 10:121–34.

Worsley A, Baghurst KI, Leitch DR. 1984. Social desirability response bias and dietary inventory responses. *Hum Nutr Appl Nutr* 38:29–35.

Yudkin JS. 1996. How to deal with regression to the mean in intervention studies. *Lancet* 347:241–243.

Zhang J, Savitz DA. 1996. Exercise during pregnancy among U.S. women. *Ann Epidemiol* 6:53–59.

Zizza C, Siega-Riz AM, Popkin BM. 2001. Significant increase in young adults' snacking between 1977–1978 and 1994–1996 represents a cause for concern. *Prev Med* 32:303–310.

A

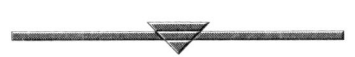

Allowed Nutrition Risk Criteria

ANTHROPOMETRIC
100   *Low Weight for Height*
101   Pre-pregnancy Underweight
102   Postpartum Underweight
103   Underweight or At Risk of Becoming Underweight (Infants and Children)*

110   *High Weight for Height*
111   Pre-pregnancy Overweight
112   Postpartum Overweight
113   Overweight (Children 2–5 years of Age)*
114   At Risk of Becoming Overweight (Infants and Children)*

120   *Short Stature*
121   Short Stature (infants, children)

130   *Inappropriate Growth/Weight Gain Pattern*
131   Low Maternal Weight Gain*
132   Maternal Weight Loss During Pregnancy
133   High Maternal Weight Gain*
134   Failure to Thrive
135   Inadequate Growth

140	*Low Birth Weight/Premature Birth*
141	Low Birth Weight
142	Prematurity

150	*Other Anthropometric Risk*
151	Small for Gestational Age
152	Low Head Circumference
153	Large for Gestational Age

BIOCHEMICAL

200	*Hematocrit or Hemoglobin Below State Criteria*
201	Low Hematocrit/Low Hemoglobin [formerly entitled Anemia]

210	*Other Biochemical Test Results Which Indicate Nutritional Abnormality*
211	Elevated Blood Lead Levels

CLINICAL/HEALTH/MEDICAL

300	*Pregnancy-Induced Conditions*
301	Hyperemesis Gravidarum
302	Gestational Diabetes
303	History of Gestational Diabetes

310	*Delivery of Low-Birthright/Premature Infant*
311	History of Preterm Delivery
312	History of Low Birthweight

320	*Prior Stillbirth, Fetal, or Neonatal Death*
321	History of Spontaneous Abortion, Fetal or Neonatal Loss

330	*General Obstetrical Risks*
331	Pregnancy at a Young Age
332	Closely Spaced Pregnancies
333	High Parity and Young Age
334	Lack of Adequate Prenatal Care
335	Multifetal Gestation
336	Fetal Growth Restriction
337	History of Birth of a Large for Gestational Age Infant
338	Pregnant Woman Currently Breastfeeding
339	History of Birth with Nutrition-Related Congenital or Birth Defect

340	*Nutrition-Related Risk Conditions (e.g.. Chronic Disease, Genetic Disorder Infection)*
341	Nutrient Deficiency Diseases
342	Gastro-Intestinal Disorders

APPENDIX A 161

343   Diabetes Mellitus
344   Thyroid Disorders
345   Hypertension (Includes Chronic and Pregnancy Induced)
346   Renal Disease
347   Cancer
348   Central Nervous System Disorders
349   Genetic and Congenital Disorders
350   Pyloric Stenosis
351   Inborn Errors of Metabolism
352   Infectious Diseases (Bronchiolitis added)
353   Food Allergies
354   Celiac Disease
355   Lactose Intolerance
356   Hypoglycemia
357   Drug-Nutrient Interactions
358   Eating Disorders
359   Recent Major Surgery, Trauma, Burns
360   Other Medical Conditions
361   Depression
362   Developmental, Sensory, or Motor Disabilities Interfering with the Ability to Eat

370   *Substance Abuse (Drugs, Alcohol, Tobacco)*
371   Maternal Smoking
372   Alcohol and Illegal Drug Use

380   *Other Health Risks*
381   Dental Problems
382   Fetal Alcohol Syndrome

DIETARY
400   *Inadequate/Inappropriate Nutrient Intake*
401   Failure to Meet USDA/DHHS Dietary Guidelines for Americans
402   Vegan Diets
403   Highly Restrictive Diets

410   *Other Dietary Risk*
411   Inappropriate Infant Feeding
412   Early Introduction of Solid Foods
413   Feeding Cow's Milk During First 12 Months
414   No Dependable Source of Iron for Infants at 6 Months of Age or Later
415   Improper Dilution of Formula
416   Feeding Other Foods Low in Essential Nutrients
417   Lack of Sanitation in Preparation/Handling of Nursing Bottles

418	Infrequent Breastfeeding as Sole Source of Nutrients
419	Inappropriate Use of Nursing Bottles
420	Excessive Caffeine Intake (Breastfeeding Women)
421	Pica
422	Inadequate Diet
423	Inappropriate or Excessive Intake of Dietary Supplements Including Vitamins, Minerals and Herbal Remedies
424	Inadequate Vitamin/Mineral Supplementation
425	Inappropriate Feeding Practices for Children
426	Inadequate Folic Acid Intake to Prevent NTD's, Spina Bifida and Anencephaly

OTHER RISKS

500	*Regression/Transfer/Presumptive Eligibility*
501	Possibility of Regression
502	Transfer of Certification
503	Presumptive Eligibility for Pregnant Women
600	*Breastfeeding Mother/Infant Dyad*
601	Breastfeeding Mother of Infant at Nutritional Risk
602	Breastfeeding Complications (Women)
603	Breastfeeding Complications (Infants)
700	*Infant of a WIC-Eligible Mother or Mother at Risk During Pregnancy*
701	Infant Up to 6 Months Old of WIC Mother, or of a Woman Who Would Have Been Eligible During Pregnancy
702	Breastfeeding Infant of Woman at Nutritional Risk
703	Infant Born of Woman with Mental Retardation or Alcohol or Drug Abuse During Most Recent Pregnancy
800	*Homelessness/Migrancy*
801	Homelessness
802	Migrancy
900	*Other Nutritional Risks*
901	Recipient of Abuse
902	Woman, or Infant/Child of Primary Caregiver with Limited Ability to Make Feeding Decisions and/or Prepare Food
903	Foster Care

*Added/modified per RISC deliberations as of March 2001.

B

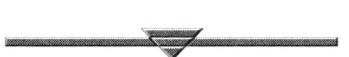

Workshop Agenda and Presentations

**Workshop on
Dietary Risk Assessment in the WIC Program**

Thursday, June 1, 2000
National Academy of Sciences
Lecture Room
2101 Constitution Avenue, N.W., Washington D.C.

8:00 a.m.   Welcome and Introduction
            Virginia Stallings, Chair

8:15   Overview of WIC Operational Issues and Practices which may
            Impact on the Selection of Dietary Risk Assessment Methodology
            Jean Anliker, University of Maryland

8:45   Overview of Assessing Adequacy of Intake: Reliability and
            Sources of Error
            Valerie Tarasuk, University of Toronto

9:30	Development of the Dietary Guidelines and their Application to the WIC Population *Cutberto Garza, Cornell University*
10:00	Development of the Food Guide Pyramid and its Application to the WIC Population *Kristin Marcoe, U.S. Department of Agriculture*
10:30	Break
10:45	Assessing Individuals' Total Food Intake and Cognitive Aspects of Questionnaires *Amy Subar, National Cancer Institute*
11:30	Use of the Block Questionnaire in the WIC Program *Gladys Block, University of California, Berkeley*
12:15 p.m.	Lunch
1:00	Use of the Harvard Food Frequency Questionnaire in the WIC Population *Graham Colditz, Harvard School of Public Health*
1:45	Assessing Dietary Intake and Risk During Pregnancy and Special Considerations in Evaluating Intake in the Hispanic Population *Anna Maria Siega-Riz, University of North Carolina*
2:30	Break
2:45	Practical Issues in the Use of Various Tools in WIC Settings *Jill Leppert, North Dakota State Department of Health;* *Amanda Watkins, Arizona Department of Health Services;* *Ann Barone, Rhode Island Department of Health;* *Carol Rankin, Mississippi Department of Health*
3:45	The Role of WIC in Assistance to the Poor and Food Insecurity as a Predictor of Dietary Risk *Bob Greenstein, Center on Budget and Policy Priorities; Lynn Parker, Food Research and Action Center*
4:30	Open Discussion and Comments
5:30	Adjourn

C

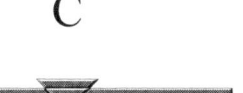

Biographical Sketches of Committee Members

VIRGINIA A. STALLINGS, M.D. *(chair)*, Chief, Nutrition Section, Division of Gastroenterology and Nutrition and Deputy Director of the Stokes Institute, The Children's Hospital of Philadelphia, and Professor of Pediatrics, the University of Pennsylvania School of Medicine. Dr. Stallings, a member of the Food and Nutrition Board, has expertise in both pediatrics and nutrition science. Dr. Stallings holds a B.S. in Nutrition and Foods from Auburn University, an M.S. in Human Nutrition and Biochemistry from Cornell University, and an M.D. degree from the University of Alabama School of Medicine. Dr. Stallings has also served as the chairperson for the Food and Nutrition Board's Committee on Nutrition Services for Medicare Beneficiaries.

TOM BARANOWSKI, PH.D., is Professor of Behavioral Nutrition, Children's Nutrition Research Center, Department of Pediatrics, Baylor College of Medicine. Dr. Baranowski earned a B.A. in politics from Princeton University and an M.A. and Ph.D. in social psychology from the University of Kansas. Dr. Baranowski's research interests are in dietary assessment procedures, intervention activities with interactive multimedia, and using the Internet to encourage dietary and physical activity behavior change.

RONETTE BRIEFEL, DR.P.H., R.D., is Senior Fellow, Mathematica Policy Research, Inc. She earned a B.S. in Nutrition from Pennsylvania State University, and an M.P.H. in Maternal and Child Health Administration and a Dr.P.H. in Epidemiology from the University of Pittsburgh's Graduate School of Public

Health. Dr. Briefel's research interests include national nutrition policy, survey research on the dietary, food security, nutritional, and health status of the U.S. population, and dietary intake methodology. She has analyzed National Health and Nutrition Examination Survey (NHANES) data on the dietary intake and nutritional status of low-income populations, including pregnant women and children participating in WIC. Dr. Briefel is a member of the American Society for Nutritional Sciences, the American Society for Clinical Nutrition, and the American Public Health Association.

YVONNE BRONNER, SC.D., R.D., L.D., is Professor and the Director of the M.P.H./Dr.P.H. Program at Morgan State University. Dr. Bronner earned a B.S. from the University of Akron, an M.S.P.H. from Case Western Reserve University, and an Sc.D. in Maternal and Child Health from Johns Hopkins School of Hygiene and Public Health. Dr. Bronner's research interests include the nutrition assessment of school children, including internal and external environment and breastfeeding promotion among African American women, and the epidemiological investigation of African American dietary knowledge, attitudes, beliefs, and practices. Early in Dr. Bronner's career, she served as a WIC nutritionist.

LAURA E. CAULFIELD, PH.D., is Associate Professor, Center for Human Nutrition and Division of Human Nutrition, Department of International Health, the Johns Hopkins School of Hygiene and Public Health. Dr. Caulfield earned a B.S. in Human Nutrition from Colorado State University and a Ph.D. in International Nutrition from Cornell University. Dr. Caulfield's research interests are in areas of maternal and infant nutrition including the role of maternal and fetal nutrition in influencing parturition, labor and delivery consequences for the mother and newborn, and the role of appropriate feeding for the postnatal growth and development of infants and children.

EZRA C. DAVIDSON, JR., M.D., is Associate Dean, Primary Care and Professor (and former chair 1971–96), Department of Obstetrics and Gynecology, Charles R. Drew University of Medicine and Science. He earned a B.S. from Morehouse College and a M.D. degree from Meharry Medical College. Dr. Davidson has had an active career in research, education and clinical and public services. He was an early contributor to the development of the technology of fetoscopy and fetal blood sampling. His research interests include fetal research and policy, adolescent pregnancy, and biomedical ethics related to reproduction. Dr. Davidson has been a member of the Institute of Medicine since 1991.

THERESA O. SCHOLL, PH.D., M.P.H., is Professor, Department of Obstetrics and Gynecology, University of Medicine and Dentistry of New Jersey, School of Medicine. Dr. Scholl earned a B.A. at Immaculata College, an M.P.H.

in epidemiology and biostatistics from Columbia University, and a Ph.D. from Temple University. Her research interests include nutrition and gestational weight gain related to pregnancy outcomes and adolescent pregnancy. She is a member of the American College of Epidemiology.

CAROL WEST SUITOR, D.SC., R.D., is a nutrition consultant working out of Northfield, Vermont. Currently, she is assisting the March of Dimes' Task Force for Nutrition and Optimal Human Development. In recent years, she served as a study director for the Food and Nutrition Board of the Institute of Medicine and as project director for the National Center for Education in Maternal and Child Health. Dr. Suitor holds a B.S. from Cornell University, an M.S. from the University of California at Berkeley, and an Sc.M. and Sc.D. from Harvard School of Public Health. Her doctoral research at the Harvard School of Public Health focused on nutrition screening for low-income pregnant women. She occasionally consults on dietary assessment methods for the Harvard group. Dr. Suitor is a member of the American Dietetic Association, the American Public Health Association, and the Society for Nutrition Education.

ROBERT WHITAKER, M.D., M.P.H., is Associate Professor of Pediatrics, Division of General and Community Pediatrics, University of Cincinnati College of Medicine, Cincinnati Children's Hospital Medical Center. Dr. Whitaker's research interests focus on childhood antecedents of adult chronic disease with particular interest in the area of childhood obesity. He earned a B.S. in chemistry at Williams College, an M.D. from the Johns Hopkins University School of Medicine and an M.P.H. from the University of Washington School of Public Health and Community Medicine.